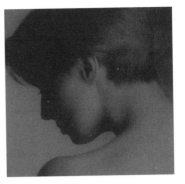

*your*
# BODY

*your*
# BEAUTY

*your*
# SAFETY

## Joseph M. Gryskiewicz, MD, FACS

*Bella*
*Surgica*

# Book Achievement Award

*Your Body, Your Beauty, Your Safety*
won First Place in the Health/Fitness/Diet/Medicine category
at the 17th Annual Midwest Independent Publishers Association (MIPA).

This book is dedicated, with deep affection, to gravity.

The information contained in this book represents the opinions of the author and should by no means be construed as a substitute for the advice of a qualified medical professional. The information contained in this book is for general reference and is intended to offer the user general information of interest. The information is not intended to replace or serve as a substitute for any medical or professional consultation or service. Certain content may represent Dr. Gryskiewicz's opinions based on his training, experience, and observation; other physicians may have differing opinions.

All information is provided "as is" and "as available" without warranties of any kind, expressed or implied, including accuracy, timeliness, and completeness. In no instance should a user attempt to diagnose a medical condition or determine appropriate treatment based on the information contained in this book. If you are experiencing any sort of medical problem or are considering cosmetic or reconstructive surgery, you should base any and all decisions only on the advice of your personal physician who has examined you and entered into a physician-patient relationship with you.

ISBN 10: 1-59298-138-0
ISBN 13: 978-1-59298-138-0

Library of Congress Catalog Number: 2006920442
Printed in Canada
First Printing: February 2006
Second Printing: 2008
Third Printing: 2014

17   16   15   14            6   5   4   3

Cover and interior design by KantorGroup, www.KantorGroup.com
Front cover photography by Douglas Beasley, www.beasleyphotography.com
Back cover portrait photography of Dr. Joe by Marie Ketring

Beaver's Pond Press, Inc.
7108 Ohms Lane
Edina, MN 55439-2129
952-829-8818
www.BeaversPondPress.com

BEAVER'S
POND
PRESS

To order, visit www.tcplasticsurgery.com
or call Bookhouse Fulfillment at 1-800-901-3480. Reseller discounts available.

# Contents

Foreword . . . . . . . . . . . . . . . . . . . . . . . . . . . . . . . . . . . . . . . . . . . . . . . . . vii

Acknowledgements . . . . . . . . . . . . . . . . . . . . . . . . . . . . . . . . . . . . . . ix

About Dr. Joe . . . . . . . . . . . . . . . . . . . . . . . . . . . . . . . . . . . . . . . . . . . xi

Introduction . . . . . . . . . . . . . . . . . . . . . . . . . . . . . . . . . . . . . . . . . . . . . 1

## PART 1: THE BASICS

**Chapter 1**    Is Plastic Surgery Right for You? . . . . . . . . . . . . . . . . . 4

**Chapter 2**    Understanding Medical Titles, Certifications,
Qualifications, and Specialties . . . . . . . . . . . . . . . . . . . . . . . . 10

**Chapter 3**    How to Choose a Cosmetic Surgeon:
A Foolproof Method . . . . . . . . . . . . . . . . . . . . . . . . . . . . . . 18

**Chapter 4**    How to Be a Terrific Patient, and Get Everything
You Want from a Plastic Surgeon . . . . . . . . . . . . . . . . . . . . 32

**Chapter 5**    Doctor and Patient Relationships . . . . . . . . . . . . . . . . . 44

## PART 2: PROCEDURES

**Chapter 6**    Breast Surgeries . . . . . . . . . . . . . . . . . . . . . . . . . . . . . . . . 50

**Chapter 7**    Rhinoplasty, Facelifts, and Other Facial Procedures . . . . . . . . . 98

**Chapter 8**    Body Work . . . . . . . . . . . . . . . . . . . . . . . . . . . . . . . . . . . . . 148

**Chapter 9**    Plastic Surgery for Men . . . . . . . . . . . . . . . . . . . . . . . . . . 176

**Chapter 10**   Revising Plastic Surgery . . . . . . . . . . . . . . . . . . . . . . . . . 182

**Chapter 11**   Taking Care of Your Skin . . . . . . . . . . . . . . . . . . . . . . . . 196

**Chapter 12**   The Rest of the Health and Beauty Picture . . . . . . . . . . . 202

**Chapter 13**   *The Zone Diet* . . . . . . . . . . . . . . . . . . . . . . . . . . . . . . . . . 216

**Chapter 14**   Frequently Asked Questions . . . . . . . . . . . . . . . . . . . . . . 222

Glossary . . . . . . . . . . . . . . . . . . . . . . . . . . . . . . . . . . . . . . . . . . . . . . 258

References . . . . . . . . . . . . . . . . . . . . . . . . . . . . . . . . . . . . . . . . . . . . 281

Index . . . . . . . . . . . . . . . . . . . . . . . . . . . . . . . . . . . . . . . . . . . . . . . . . 283

# Foreword

Thousands of Americans turn to plastic surgery each year as the ultimate makeover program. Unfortunately, their decisions are often made without having the necessary information. This is why this book is so important as it answers many of the questions that should be asked before embarking on plastic surgery.

However, as Dr. Joe Gryskiewicz points out, the benefits of plastic surgery can become dramatically enhanced by paying careful attention to the diet, and specifically *The Zone Diet*. Make no mistake about it. Plastic surgery represents a significant stress to the body. Preparing the body to handle that stress, reduce recovery times, and sustain the benefits is accomplished through the diet. I have worked with Dr. Joe for many years on using diet to improve surgical outcomes. This is why I would describe Dr. Joe's philosophy as *integrative* plastic surgery. More importantly, the same dietary program to maximize the external enhancement of physical appearance that can be achieved through plastic surgery will simultaneously increase the internal beauty of the body by increasing the wellness of the patient. This represents a true makeover in reversing the aging process that is the primary driving force behind most plastic surgery.

Ultimately this book is about good medicine, and that is a two-way street. The patient has to take responsibility for their future as well as being knowledgeable about any procedure being recommended to them. Dr. Joe is able to combine these two into a very readable book that allows the potential patient to obtain the ultimate rewards that *integrative* plastic surgery has to offer.

Dr. Barry Sears
Zone Laboratories, Inc.
Author of *The Zone*

# Acknowledgements

I'd like to thank my wife, Clarice, and my mother, Phyllis. Kudos also go to Bryn Collins, Mary Dahlen, Paula Hanegraaf Kenow, Michelle Kearney, Melanie Morrison, Jessica McMillan, and Mary Russell for helping to prepare this manuscript. An individual thanks goes to Mary Russell who made the manuscript easy to read.

I am grateful to each and every one of my wonderful patients who have trusted me over the years. I give a special thanks to those select patients who graciously allowed me to use their photos in this book.

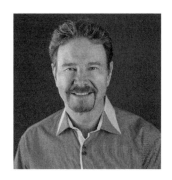

# About Dr. Joe

Joe Gryskiewicz, MD, FACS, (pronounced Gris-Kă´-vitz) has practiced medicine in the Twin Cities of Minneapolis and St. Paul for more than twenty years. He is a Clinical Professor at the University of Minnesota Cleft Palate Clinics School of Dentistry and is past Chief of Surgery at Fairview Southdale Hospital in the Minneapolis suburb of Edina. His practice, Gryskiewicz Twin Cities Cosmetic Surgery, has offices in Edina and Burnsville, Minnesota.

Dr. Gryskiewicz graduated from the University of St. Thomas in St. Paul, Minnesota, in 1972 with a bachelor's degree in nursing through the registered nursing program at the College of St. Catherine. He graduated from the University of Minnesota medical school in 1978. His post-graduate medical training included seven years of surgical residency at the University of Wisconsin Health Sciences Center.

Dr. Gryskiewicz is certified by the American Board of Plastic Surgery and received a certificate of special training in cosmetic surgery from the American Society for Aesthetic Plastic Surgery (ASAPS). He has been an official spokesperson for the American Society of Plastic Surgeons (ASPS). He is Chairman of the Emerging Trends Task Force, and belongs to numerous professional organizations and committees, including ASAPSs/ASPSs Innovative Procedures Committee. As a moderator for its biannual Hot Topics in Plastic Surgery course, he keeps up on cutting-edge developments in his field. He is an active member of the Rhinoplasty Society and serves on its committees. He also holds several issued patents for surgical devices. Dr. Gryskiewicz was inducted into the International Society of Clinical Plastic Surgeons in 2003.

Although he has extensive training in all aspects of cosmetic and plastic surgery, Dr. Gryskiewicz's special medical interests are breast augmentation, nose surgery, facial plastic surgery, and body contouring. He was one of the early adopters of suction-assisted lipectomy after studying with Dr. Simon Fredricks of Houston, Texas in 1984. Dr. Fredricks was one of the first plastic surgeons to perform liposuction.

Dr. Gryskiewicz speaks internationally and has given over one hundred presentations to professional organizations on topics such as breast augmentation and nose surgery. He writes regularly for numerous medical journals and other publications, and is a guest reviewer for the international journals *Aesthetic Surgery Journal* and the *Journal of Plastic and Reconstructive Surgery.*

Dr. Joseph Gryskiewicz was inspired to pursue a career in plastic surgery after a six-month trip as a volunteer in San Lucas Tolimán, Guatemala. Journeying by Jeep to the remote, guerrilla-occupied mountain regions, he worked around the clock, seven days a week, treating patients plagued with parasites, malnutrition, and tuberculosis. His most moving experiences came while living at the *Casa Feliz* orphanage, where he worked with the Cachchequal tribe of Central American Mayan Indians. Many of the orphans suffered from cleft lips or palates, and the life-changing difference a simple procedure made for them altered Dr. Gryskiewicz's life as well.

He and his family are devoted to assisting the people of Third World countries. His heartwarming, electrifying adventures with the Cachchequal Mayan Indians, as well as other medical journeys, will be featured in his upcoming book, tentatively titled *Three Faces.*

Dr. Gryskiewicz travels annually to South America with the international aid organizations *Interplast* and *San Francisco de Asis* to operate on children with cleft lips, cleft palates, and burns. This work is featured in the book, *Caring Hands: Inspiring Stories of Volunteer Medical Missions* by Susan I. Alexis, in the chapter "Correcting the Negative." For this and other volunteer work, he received the WCCO Radio Good Neighbor Award in 1986 and the University of St. Thomas Humanitarian of the Year Award in 1992. *Minneapolis St. Paul Magazine* has named him one of the area's Top Doctors and he has been quoted in *Elle* and *Allure* magazines.

Dr. Gryskiewicz lives in Minneapolis with his wife and enjoys art, photography, composing music, and cross-country skiing. An avid runner and triathlon competitor, Dr. Gryskiewicz has completed the Twin Cities, Boston, New York, and Chicago marathons, as well as Minnesota's Liberty Triathlon, a half iron man competition. He also took first place in his age group in the 2008 Chisago Lakes Triathlon half iron man distance.

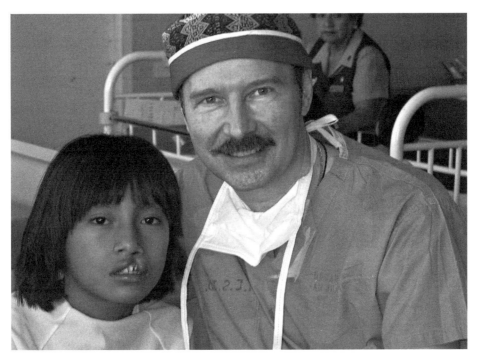

Dr. Joe with a young cleft lip patient in Lima, Peru. She told him, "I want to put lipstick on two lips rather than three."

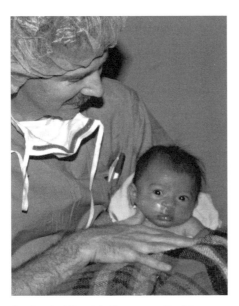

Dr. Joe holding his three-month-old bilateral cleft lip patient as she wakes up from anesthesia.

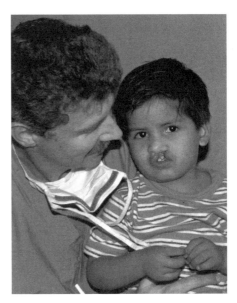

Dr. Joe sits with a little friend waiting for cleft lip repair in Guayquil, Ecuador.

# Introduction

Patients often ask if I am artistic. I tell them that in grade school, I was excused from normal class to draw wall murals of current study topics from history, social studies, etc. I sat at my desk and drew or painted all day while my classmates studied less interesting subjects and resented me.

The *plastic* in plastic surgery comes from the Greek word *plasticos*, meaning "to shape, mold, or form." I consider myself an artist as much as a surgeon. I loved general surgery, but it wasn't as personal or as artistic as plastic surgery. Restoring a patient with a serious deformity to a more normal appearance is very fulfilling, but helping rebuild someone's self-esteem holds the most meaning for me. There's a different kind of excitement in adding something to a person's life. That's what gets me up in the morning.

This book is meant for busy people who want a quick, readable source of information on cosmetic surgery. Other surgeons will have other opinions, lots of opinions. This guide isn't meant to be the cosmetic surgery gospel according to Dr. Joe—just a friendly reference with essential tidbits of information to help you make a decision about cosmetic surgery that's right for you.

Dr. Joe Gryskiewicz

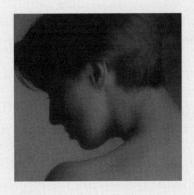

# Part 1: The Basics

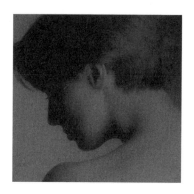

*chapter 1*

# IS PLASTIC SURGERY
# RIGHT FOR YOU?

"It's good to have an end to journey toward,

but it is the journey that matters in the end."

— Author Ursula K. LeGuin

*O*ne day, you look in the mirror and say to yourself, "That's it, I'm doing it." Maybe it's that bump on your nose you've been looking at for twenty years. Maybe it's your breasts, which once did full justice to your favorite bikini but now are facing due south after you've had three kids. Or maybe it's those bags under your eyes that make you look tired no matter how awake and energized you feel.

According to the most recent statistics from the American Society for Aesthetic Plastic Surgery (ASAPS), the number of surgeries performed jumped 465 percent from 1997 through 2004. Nearly 11.9 million cosmetic procedures were performed in 2004 alone. ASAPS statistics show women had 92 percent of the procedures while men had eight percent.

Baby boomers between the ages of 35 and 50 had the most cosmetic surgery procedures in 2002—45 percent, while 19 to 34 year olds had 24 percent of procedures, and 51 through 64 year olds had 22 percent. People 65 and older had only six percent of cosmetic surgery overall, and people under 18 had only three percent.

Among U.S. women, 55 percent say they approve of cosmetic surgery, and 54 percent of men agree. The higher a person's income and education, the higher the approval rating.

Deciding to have a surgical procedure is a balancing act between your expectations, wishes, dreams and reality. Realizing what to expect is half the battle. Keep this essential truth in mind: Gravity always wins. Even though you have a facelift, you will continue to age. Here's what I tell prospective facelift patients: Pretend you have an identical twin who will not have the surgery. You'll both continue to age normally, but you will always look about seven years younger.

Is it unhealthy for people to be unhappy with what God gave them? I don't believe it is. I believe that the goal of plastic surgery should not be to change my patients' basic appearance, but to prevent them from looking older than they need to and to enhance their body image, elevating their self-esteem. It's like living in a beautiful older home. It's only beautiful because it's kept in good repair. If the porch sags, I fix it. Why treat your body with any less care?

*"In you, I saw a professional artist and doctor,"* one of my patients wrote. *"It was clear you wanted to see a nice change, not dramatic, but a change to fit me. My family and people I work with think I look terrific and can't put their*

*finger on just why. But I didn't have my surgery for anyone but me. It is private, yet I have this never-ending grin on my face all of the time."*

Isn't plastic surgery frivolous? I don't think so. I've seen so many patients energized by a rejuvenating surgical procedure. My goal is to help people be happy with their appearance and improve how they feel about themselves.

*"Surgery altered my outlook as much as my appearance,"* according to one patient. *"It was as if I had dropped 20 years and a lifetime of abuse and hard times, and finally discovered that I deserved a good life."*

Another patient, newly married, described how nose surgery and a chin implant changed her self-concept, giving her confidence to pose for wedding pictures. It was the most significant thing she had done in her entire life, this patient wrote.

One breast-reduction patient from many years ago couldn't work because of back, neck, and shoulder pain. She had been on welfare and received disability payments. Following surgery, her social worker called to report she had taken on a new job and had a "new life" because of the breast reduction.

Another patient—who had nose surgery, a chin implant, a facelift, earlobe reduction, and a tummy tuck—wrote:

*"Since my surgeries, weekly or more often someone comments on how good I'm looking. I just smile and say 'thank you.' On a recent anniversary trip, one woman guessed my age as 15 years younger than I am. These compliments motivate me to continue my exercise program, as well as other healthy life choices. I want to be around for my family for as long as possible."*

Also consider the effect cosmetic surgery can have on the self-esteem of a child taunted for having a physical abnormality. During medical training, I saw a 12-year-old boy from rural Wisconsin who had protruding ears—the other kids called him Dumbo. To fix the problem, his father had applied Superglue behind each ear. This worked, but several weeks later a foul odor developed. When I examined the boy in the emergency room, I could see that the skin behind each ear had died, exposing the actual cartilage framework. This young boy needed subsequent skin grafting and eventually did well, but he could have been spared a lot of suffering if he had had cosmetic surgery in the first place.

*"I didn't see the real me when I looked in the mirror,"* one patient wrote. *"I wasn't ready to accept where my physical outward appearance was placing me. I decided to seek alternatives. I had a facelift, eyelid tuck, and fat injection. Now my outside me reflects my energy and joy of life and no longer makes me look tired and older than my spirit."*

Plastic surgery isn't dieting, exercise, or other forms of self-improvement. It does expose you to a certain amount of health risk. Plastic surgery is no different from any other operation in that respect, although the vast majority of cosmetic procedures have a low rate of complications. For people who place a high priority on appearance or are adversely affected by their self-image, the benefits of plastic surgery can greatly outweigh the risks.

Many patients are set on proceeding with surgery even before I consult with them. Others take a lot more time to make up their minds. If you are ambivalent, come back for a second visit or call your surgeon on the phone to review your situation as many times as you need to.

That's how I handle my practice. You might think of twenty questions while you are driving home. "Write them all down," I instruct my patients. "Then call me on the phone or come in for a second visit if you want clarification. We'll go through your list until all your questions are answered."

## COSMETIC SURGERY INFORMATION ON-LINE

One of the best ways to make up your mind about cosmetic surgery is to surf the web. I'm continually amazed at the detailed information about cosmetic surgery available on the Internet. Patients who consult me about breast augmentation want to review Internet photos of rippling, asymmetry, visible contour problems, and size issues. Web cruisers are the most informed consumers I encounter in my practice. It's easy to be overwhelmed with too much information, but the extensive detail available on-line is invaluable.

Gryskiewicz Twin Cities Cosmetic Surgery's website can be found at **www.tcplasticsurgery.com.** Good sites for breast implant information are **www.implantinfo.com** and **www.lookingyourbest.com.** Additional information online can be found at www.plasticsurgery.org. Another informative website, www.makemeheal.com, focuses on recovery issues, symptoms, prevention and treatment of complications, and risks. You can access the homepage, but need to subscribe to the various programs.

## REASONS NOT TO HAVE PLASTIC SURGERY

Whatever the body part, whatever the reason, you've resolved that cosmetic surgery is the answer. But is it? Just because you've decided you want to have a procedure done doesn't mean you should. For every reason to have cosmetic surgery, there are reasons not to.

Here are some good reasons not to have plastic surgery:

- To please your spouse or partner.
- As a reaction to a midlife crisis.
- As a reaction to a life-changing event, such as a death or divorce.
- If you suffer from ongoing depression.
- If you have any major health problems.
- To land "Mr. Wonderful."
- To just "be happy."

Some patients tell me they've decided not to have surgery because their friends don't want them to change. Your friends shouldn't unduly influence your decision, but if you believe they are an important part of the equation, then perhaps you should opt out. Don't undergo a rejuvenating surgical procedure to save your marriage. The procedure will never meet your expectations. Nor will an eyelid tuck and a hair transplant guarantee that an aging male will land a job promotion. You need to be sure your reasons for having surgery are realistic.

A good plastic surgeon is going to look at any of the above reasons as red flags. If the surgeon has compassion and ethics, he or she will turn you away gently until the issues in your life are resolved. That doesn't mean you'll never get the procedure you want, but when you do decide to go ahead, it will be for the right reasons.

You also should avoid plastic surgery if you're a perfectionist and want guaranteed results; if you feel the need for multiple preoperative consultations and still feel indecisive; or if your intuition simply tells you "no." Sometimes you also have to listen to your doctor. If a plastic surgeon says he or she can't do what you've requested or doesn't believe your request will enhance your appearance, maybe surgery isn't right for you.

If none of the above applies to you, you're probably ready to have the cosmetic surgery you want. Read on. There's a wealth of information here, and there's a lot you need to know, even before setting foot in a doctor's office.

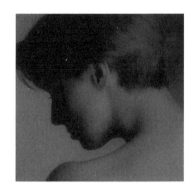

*chapter 2*

# UNDERSTANDING MEDICAL TITLES, CERTIFICATIONS, QUALIFICATIONS, AND SPECIALTIES

"We get most of our exercise jumping to conclusions."

– Anonymous

osmetic surgery may seem like forbidden fruit because it's what your health insurance doesn't cover. The investigation process doesn't start by flipping through your HMO manual. You have to do your homework. Beyond financial considerations are far more important issues. You don't want to have unreasonable expectations, too much surgery, or end up having a procedure done by a podiatrist who happened to buy a laser and advertises himself as a cosmetic surgeon. This chapter will help you understand a surgeon's training and qualifications.

## BOARD CERTIFICATION

Many consumers are utterly baffled when it comes to board certification. They confuse it with state licensing. Others think the American Medical Association certifies plastic surgeons. Some consumers have a vague idea that surgeons specialize after receiving their medical degrees, but have no idea how this training differs from that received by those who call themselves cosmetic surgeons.

A doctor of medicine, or M.D., degree is given at graduation from an accredited medical school. Once an M.D. degree is achieved, a license must be obtained from the state where a physician desires to practice. This state license allows an M.D. to practice in any specialty whatsoever, regardless of training beyond the M.D. degree. After receiving a medical degree, most physicians enroll in a residency program, which gives them expertise in a particular area. Following this training, they can take another examination given by a medical specialty board (called "boards") and become certified in that particular specialty. So, a medical degree, a state license, and board certification are three different qualifications.

Currently, any licensed physician is legally allowed to perform cosmetic surgery procedures. In fact, if you have M.D. after your name you can even do brain surgery, whether you have any surgical training or not. Scary, isn't it? I could legally perform brain surgery. Just think, an untrained, left-handed, Polish brain surgeon.

What would prevent a physician from doing this? Well, some insurance companies won't allow a surgeon to be on their rosters unless they're board certified. Hospitals restrict privileges unless appropriate training can be documented. A lot of cosmetic surgery is done in private offices or in surgery centers, so people can call themselves "cosmetic surgeons" without hospital privileges and credibility in the professional community.

The increased number of physicians without plastic surgery training who are performing cosmetic procedures directly correlates with the advent of managed care and the consequent decrease in physician income. Some physicians view cosmetic surgery—paid for by the patient and outside the control of managed care—as a way to recover lost income. We call these doctors "skimmers." They don't want to put in the long hours required for surgical training, but they do want to skim the profits off this potentially lucrative branch of surgery.

You might assume that certain medical specialists are automatically trained in cosmetic surgery procedures, but this isn't necessarily the case. Ear, nose, and throat specialists, for example, may not be trained to do cosmetic rhinoplasty (nose jobs). Some have taken additional surgical training and do perform cosmetic facial plastic surgery. Others shy away from cosmetic procedures and specialize in nasal airway reconstruction or other non-cosmetic surgeries. Many ear, nose, and throat (ENT) surgeons do excellent cosmetic facial surgery, but it isn't part of their specialty's training. To be certified in facial plastic surgery, an ENT surgeon must have additional training.

When it comes to cosmetic surgery, I don't believe there needs to be a turf battle between doctors or specialties. Instead, what really matters are patient rights and safety. Patients have a right to know the full nature and extent of their doctor's formal training. Consumers can choose whatever kind of physician they wish, but they should be given the information needed to make an informed choice.

## THE PLASTIC SURGERY SPECIALTY

Plastic surgeons are trained to perform surgery. This might sound obvious, but not many consumers know that only some of the 24 medical specialties recognized by the American Board of Medical Specialties include surgical training. The Board and the American Medical Association Council on Medical Education officially approve medical specialty boards. These are in areas as diverse as allergies, immunology, and medical genetics. There are specific surgical boards for orthopedic surgery, thoracic surgery, general surgery and, of course, plastic surgery.

After medical school, plastic surgeons must complete a minimum of five years of surgical training, including a plastic surgery residency program, before they can be board certified. The training encompasses both reconstructive and cosmetic surgery procedures for both the face and the body. A good background in reconstructive surgery is excellent training for cosmetic surgery. During my general surgery training, for example, I did quite a bit of work in the burn unit. This taught me about fluid and electrolyte balance and fluid resuscitation techniques, which are often applicable when I'm doing liposuction.

Plastic surgeons are trained to prevent and handle emergencies if necessary. A comprehensive education includes a sound foundation in medicine, anatomy, and physiology that is vitally important to patient safety. With their board education, plastic surgeons have access to a wide range of treatments. They have the training to offer their patients the most suitable cosmetic procedures to fit their needs. The surgeon's recommendations are enhanced by training and ability to obtain hospital privileges to perform complex procedures when necessary.

A plastic surgeon's training develops both technical skills and aesthetic judgment. The experience gained through years of doing complex reconstructive surgery provides plastic surgeons with outstanding technical skills. Additionally, the continuous attention to form as well as function provides these specialists with a finely tuned sense of aesthetics—the unique qualification critical to the success of cosmetic surgery, where an artist's sense of balance and proportion is needed. I tell each patient, "I'm an artist, trying to be a mind reader." I strive to give the customized surgical outcome each patient mentally envisions. Everyone comes with his or her own building blocks.

### The American Board of Plastic Surgery

The American Board of Plastic Surgery (ABPS) certifies plastic surgeons. The ABPS is the only board approved by the American Board of Medical Specialties and the American Medical Association council for certifying physicians in plastic surgery. ABPS's primary purpose is to evaluate and pass judgment on the training and knowledge of broadly competent plastic surgeons.

The American Board of Plastic Surgery establishes requirements for doctors seeking plastic surgery training and sets standards for graduate education in this specialty. It conducts qualifying written and oral exams for certification.

ABPS certification requires graduation from an accredited medical school and a minimum of three years of clinical training in general surgery or completion of an approved residency in neurological, orthopedic, otolaryngology (ENT), or urology surgery. This is followed by a minimum of

## Be on the Lookout for Made-up Cosmetic Surgery Boards

The American Board of Medical Specialties doesn't recognize anything called the American Board of Cosmetic Surgery, but there's a good chance you'll find it proudly cited in the classified ads in popular women's magazines. Currently, anyone can create a board and claim to be certified by it.

## What do the initials "FACS" mean?

When the initials "FACS" follow the name of a surgeon, it means the surgeon is a member of a specific surgical society: "Fellow of the American College of Surgeons"

## Web site for the American Society of Plastic Surgeons (ASPS)

www.plasticsurgery.org

two years of approved residency training in plastic surgery in the United States or Canada. Combined programs lasting six years also exist to train plastic surgeons.

### SPECIALIZING IN CONFUSION

The plastic surgery certification is a broad one, and includes both reconstructive and cosmetic surgery. There is no recognized medical specialty board that certifies anything called cosmetic surgery. There are some made-up cosmetic surgery boards, though. In fact, they would accredit my teen-aged daughter if I sent them $400. In a month she'd have a certificate on her bedroom wall right next to her rock star posters.

The American Board of Medical Specialties doesn't recognize anything called the American Board of Cosmetic Surgery, for example, but there's a good chance you'll find it proudly cited in the classified ads in popular women's magazines. Currently, anyone can create a board and claim to be certified by it. Make sure your plastic surgeon isn't accredited by the American Board of Skimmers, the American Board of I Just Bought a Laser but Really I'm a Podiatrist, or the American Board of I'll Call Myself a Cosmetic Surgeon Because State Law Protects Me and Who'll Know the Difference. Many of these self-designated boards simply don't have the checks and balances that ensure consistent, objective evaluation—or, unfortunately, any evaluation at all.

A persistent problem for cosmetic surgeons is that the public perceives board-certified plastic surgeons as generalists and assumes that doctors with subspecialty credentials are specialists, and thus more qualified. Physicians with a certificate from a weekend seminar on liposuction are seen as the equals of plastic surgeons or, worse, as the true specialists. Some plastic surgeons believe the field needs a subspecialty certificate in cosmetic surgery to help the public identify physicians who are properly trained and to ensure the competency of those claiming to be specialists in cosmetic procedures.

Other plastic surgeons believe introducing yet another certifying board will confuse the public even more. After all, we've been saying for a long time that the only valid certifying board for plastic surgery is the American Board of Plastic Surgery—do we really want to change that? So far, the American Board of Medical Specialties has been unwilling to support another board for cosmetic surgery, so there are currently no board-certified cosmetic subspecialty certificates granted in plastic surgery. As a consumer, your best choice is an ABPS certified plastic surgeon with a particular interest in cosmetic surgery.

## PROFESSIONAL ORGANIZATIONS

In addition to board certification, there are well-respected professional organizations that will only admit reputable plastic surgeons to their membership. When you are selecting a surgeon, check to see if he or she belongs to the American Society of Plastic Surgeons—almost all board-certified plastic surgeons do. And look for membership in the American Society of Aesthetic Plastic Surgery, a professional society for plastic surgeons who specialize in cosmetic procedures. It holds its members to extremely high standards.

### The American Society of Plastic Surgeons

The main organization for specialists in both reconstructive and cosmetic surgery is the American Society of Plastic Surgeons (ASPS). This society was founded in 1931 and 97 percent of all physicians certified by the American Board of Plastic Surgery are members. The society's purpose is to educate the public about plastic surgery, both aesthetic and reconstructive, and to assist individuals in selecting a properly trained and experienced physician.

The organization promotes research and high professional standards of care through scientific education and acts as an advocate with the government and insurance industry. It offers practice management services and coordinates

## Where Can You Check a Surgeon's Credentials?

### The American Society for Aesthetic Plastic Surgery (ASAPS)

The society encourages prospective patients to make informed choices by investigating the credentials of any physician they are considering for their cosmetic surgery. It's a good idea to call them when you're looking for or researching a plastic surgeon. The phone number is 888-ASAPS-11.

### American Board of Medical Specialists (ABMS)

This web-based service found at www.abms.org allows the public to verify FREE OF CHARGE the board certification status, location by city and state and specialty of any physician certified by one or more of the 24 Member Boards of the ABMS.

### Contact Your State's Medical Board

A directory of state medical boards can be found at: http://www.mhsource.com/resource/board.html

similar activities. The society publishes the *Journal of Plastic and Reconstructive Surgery*, a monthly publication that contains numerous articles on reconstructive and cosmetic procedures.

ASPS members also participate in various programs to provide free reconstructive care to residents of underdeveloped nations. Members help impoverished children with cleft lips and palates, burns, and hand injuries.

### The American Society of Aesthetic Plastic Surgery

The American Society for Aesthetic Plastic Surgery (ASAPS) is the leading professional society for plastic surgeons who have been certified by the American Board of Plastic Surgery and want to further specialize in cosmetic surgery. The society encourages prospective patients to make informed choices by investigating the credentials of any physician they are considering for their cosmetic surgery. It's a good idea to call them when you're looking for or researching a plastic surgeon. The phone number is **888-ASAPS-11**.

The society's mission is to advance the science and art of cosmetic plastic surgery through support and direction of education and research, to promote the highest standards of ethical conduct and responsible patient care, and to serve the public interest by providing timely information on cosmetic plastic surgery. The society publishes the *Aesthetic Surgery Journal*, with numerous articles on cosmetic procedures, six times a year.

The ASAPS membership includes about 1,500 U.S. plastic surgeons who have been elected to join the prestigious organization. Another 1,100 are enrolled in the society's candidate program.

Among the requirements for election to membership are:
- Certification by the American Board of Plastic Surgery.
- At least three years of active practice following board certification.
- A surgical case list demonstrating an extensive number of cosmetic procedures (this stringent requirement prohibits many skilled surgeons from entering the society).
- Documented continuing medical education credits in cosmetic surgery for 36 months prior to application.
- Sponsorship by two active members.
- Submission of current marketing/advertising materials for review.
- Adherence to the society's code of ethics for professional conduct.

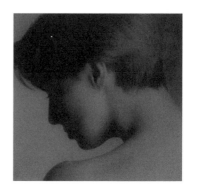

*chapter 3*

# HOW TO CHOOSE A COSMETIC SURGEON: A FOOLPROOF METHOD

"I should have done my homework

before having the procedure, I know that."

— Dissatisfied plastic surgery patient

$\mathcal{O}$K, you've made up your mind to go ahead with a consultation. How do you avoid the podiatrist who bought a laser and is advertising himself as a cosmetic surgeon? This chapter will help you find a skilled professional and artistic practitioner who is technically excellent and will meet your needs.

## USE THE YELLOW PAGES WITH DISCRETION

Don't begin, or end for that matter, with the Yellow Pages. Remember the podiatrist who bought the laser? Believe it or not, he can be listed in the Yellow Pages as a plastic surgeon. State agencies or licensing boards don't review the Yellow Pages. Physicians can call themselves plastic surgeons whether or not they've had one day of training. As I thumb through my local Yellow Pages, the first several names I read are excellent colleagues whom I know well, but buried within the list I see two dermatologists who don't have any surgical residency training for cosmetic procedures.

In fact, I saw a highly dissatisfied patient of one of the dermatologists in my office recently. The woman had wanted the deepening cheek folds on her face reduced and was livid about the six highly visible scars left behind when a synthetic material was surgically inserted to plump them up. She wanted me to fix the scars, but once skin is cut a scar is permanent. It might be improved, but it can never be erased. Once she discovered the doctor who performed the procedure was a dermatologist and not a plastic surgeon, she refused to return to him for further work. We agreed she should have done her homework before having the procedure.

Another ad I see in the Yellow Pages reads "Miracles performed daily!" Yet another, placed by a dermatologist, claims membership in the American Academy of Cosmetic Surgery. That's nice, and maybe they get together once in a while for lunch (assuming it has more than one member). But it doesn't say anything about this person's qualifications. Remember, the American Board of Plastic Surgery (ABPS) is the only board approved by the American Board of Medical Specialties and the American Medical Association to certify physicians in plastic surgery.

## FALSE ADVERTISING

Never select a plastic surgeon based on advertising alone. Cosmetic surgery is real surgery. Read physicians' advertisements with a critical eye. Be careful of advertisements that promise "painless" or "easy" surgery, guarantee results, or use language intended to persuade or mislead prospective patients. Articles from peer-reviewed journals should back up claims or promises. Ask for pertinent references; it's your right. Claims should be based on scientific studies.

One ad I noticed offered "scarless breast enlargement surgery." Sorry, but this is unrealistic. There has to be a scar somewhere. There are four approaches to breast enlargement surgery: an incision in the crease under the breast, around the rim of the nipple, or through the belly button or armpit. Surgery through the armpit could be considered almost scarless, but this is one of the common surgical options, not something unusual. This particular ad used this "fact" in an imaginative fashion to capture a prospective patient's attention. In this case a statement used for marketing purposes could easily mislead an uninformed person. Incidentally, a skilled doctor in my state does breast enlargement through the belly button, but he doesn't advertise "scarless" surgery.

Some advertising claims, such as "scarless facelift surgery," are openly deceptive. This is preposterous. All facelifts leave scars. Maybe they're talking about a "thread lift," or a chemical peel, or fat suction, or maybe they aren't talking about anything at all. They just want to get people in the front door.

Appropriate advertising will state a surgeon's credentials, including certifications from boards that actually exist. Be sure to ask about total years of training, experience, and areas of expertise, and if you feel you are getting a sales pitch instead of answers, be wary.

## BEWARE THE HYPE

Being quoted in a popular magazine, appearing on television, or speaking on the radio or at public events aren't a guarantee of a surgeon's qualifications. Some are asked because they serve as spokespeople for reputable professional organizations, but others have public relations representatives hired to obtain print or broadcast exposure. A doctor who appears in the media may be an excellent and reputable physician, but don't assume anything. Assumption is the mother of all screw-ups. Do some research beyond the hype, and find out the truth for yourself.

## SCAN WEBSITES

Websites can be a good way to get information about plastic surgery and plastic surgeons, but as with the Yellow Pages, use discretion. Anyone can have a website—whether they are skilled board certified surgeons or our podiatrist friend. The American Society of Aesthetic Plastic Surgery sponsors some excellent sites at **www.surgery.org**. You might also want to visit our website at **www.tcplasticsurgery.com** for more information on procedures and links to other sites.

There's a lot of information available on the Internet, and you can learn about the procedure you are considering. It's also nice to be able to compare the opinions you find at different sites. You can do good research without leaving your house as long as you are wary of quack sites. The more you know about the procedure you are considering, the better you will be able to evaluate the doctors you interview later.

## HEAR IT THROUGH THE GRAPEVINE

Recommendations from friends and acquaintances can help you develop a list of potential plastic surgeons. Once you've narrowed it down, talking with satisfied patients about their results is a good way to find out more. My office maintains a patient referral list that gives prospective patients the first name and phone number of patients who have volunteered to discuss their surgeries. We call this our Happy Patient List. It is the kindred-soul club of plastic surgery, and you can learn a lot from talking to others who have had a procedure you are considering (this is a great resource, but keep in mind that every person is unique, and your experience and results won't be exactly the same as anyone else's. Your surgeon should be the first to tell you that).

Remember the old ad line, "Only her hairdresser knows for sure"? Believe it or not, I receive many referrals from these informed

## Reliable Cosmetic Surgery Websites

www.surgery.org

www.plasticsurgery.org

www.breastimplantsafety.com

www.lookingyourbest.com

www.makemeheal.com

www.breastdrs.com

www.implantinfo.com

**Dr. Joe's site:**
www.tcplasticsurgery.com

professionals. After all, hairdressers are in an excellent position to evaluate how different facelift, brow-lift, and eyelid scars are hidden, and they are trained to have a good eye for aesthetics. And because they see such a variety of clients, they are also in a great position to compare the techniques of different plastic surgeons.

## ASK THE FAMILY DOCTOR

I also receive many referrals from family physicians who have seen my work, and they can be a great resource for you. Bear in mind, though, that they may have no idea whether I am technically excellent in the operating room or not. For some surgeons, everything appears easy. Watching them work with their scrub nurse is like watching a highly choreographed dance. For others, everything seems to be a struggle. Only another plastic surgeon or the operating room personnel who watch a surgeon operate could really tell patients if their choice is a plastic surgeon with "magic hands."

Your family doctor may or may not be knowledgeable when it comes to the technical skills involved in cosmetic surgery, and his or her familiarity with plastic surgeons in the community may vary widely. Listen to your family doctor's advice, but continue to gather information on your own.

## CHECK WITH PROFESSIONAL ORGANIZATIONS

Your next step should be to check with the professional organizations that deal with plastic surgery. Call the American Society of Plastic Surgeons (ASPS) physician referral service at **800-635-0635**, and within a week you will receive a list of five members who practice in your geographic area. The American Board of Plastic Surgery certifies all ASPS members. You can also call this number to find out whether a surgeon you have in mind is board certified. If you'd like to contact the American Board of Plastic Surgery directly, the number is **215-587-9322**.

Another great resource is the American Society of Aesthetic Plastic Surgery. Its members are plastic surgeons who have a particular specialty in cosmetic plastic surgery. You can call the cosmetic surgery referral line at **888-ASAPS-11** or visit their website at **www.surgery.org** to locate surgeons in your area. Use the "Find a Surgeon" locator. The site also has an abundance of useful information on cosmetic surgery procedures as well as nonsurgical techniques such as laser resurfacing and collagen injection.

## CALL YOUR STATE'S MEDICAL BOARD

Between your friends and acquaintances, your family practitioner, the American Society of Plastic Surgeons, the American Society for Aesthetic Plastic Surgery, and your hair stylist, you should have at least five plastic surgeons on your list. You can call your state's medical board to ask for current license verification and about any disciplinary action taken against your prospective surgeon.

This is a very important step. Recently, a patient handed me a full report on disciplinary actions taken against a local surgeon she had received from the state medical board. I was impressed by this woman's detective work, which was just a phone call away. This kind of information is publicly available for the asking.

State medical boards don't dispense disciplinary action lightly. A good deal of thought and investigation goes into it. Check the credentials carefully of anyone who would rearrange or reshape your body or face. In this case, paranoia is only heightened awareness.

## TALK TO SOME SURGEONS

All of this should have narrowed things down pretty well for you. Now it's time to start calling some doctors. Ask the receptionist whether the surgeon has a particular specialty, such as breast augmentation, rhinoplasty, liposuction, or facelifts. Ask about the doctor's training in that specialty. In general, for the best possible results you should look for a surgeon who specializes in the procedure you are considering, has training in that procedure, and does a lot of them. This should help you narrow things down even further.

If you're extremely comfortable with the first doctor you visit, you may decide not to seek a second opinion. As long as you've done your homework, that's fine. It's also fine to interview several different doctors before you find the right one for you. Keep in mind, though, opinions about the best techniques and procedures might differ. **If you ask five general surgeons whether a patient's diseased gallbladder needs to be removed and how, you'll probably receive a unanimous answer or close to it. If you ask five plastic surgeons how to proceed with breast augmentation, you'll likely get five different answers. Remember that plastic surgery is as much art as it is science.**

## Finding an Excellent Cosmetic Surgeon

- Familiarize yourself with physicians' qualifications, titles, and certifications.

- Use the Yellow Pages with discretion.

- Scan websites for general information.

- Learn as much as you can about the procedure you want.

- Consult friends and family who have had plastic surgery.

- Consult your family doctor.

- Don't forget your hairdresser.

- Call professional organizations like the American Society for Aesthetic Plastic Surgery or the American Society of Plastic Surgeons.

- Make a list of the names you've been given.

- Call your state's medical board to check on prospective doctors.

- Meet with the doctors.

- Choose a surgeon you trust and with whom you feel comfortable.

When you are making your appointments, pick a time toward the end of the day, if you can. From my perspective, I feel I have more time to discuss surgery with patients then because my schedule is winding down. Earlier in the day, I may be distracted knowing other patients are waiting in adjacent examination rooms. Don't dress up for the visit, but don't dress down, either. The main thing is to just be yourself. An open-minded, inquisitive attitude is your best posture at this initial visit.

### OFFICE ATMOSPHERE

Have you ever entered a business where the staff sincerely says, "Boy, you look good?" I hear my office staff say things like this to patients. From your first phone call for an appointment to your last office visit, ask yourself: Did the office staff meet my expectations? Did they make me feel good about myself? Were they courteous? Did they listen to me, or were they rushed? Did I have a modicum of privacy at the front desk, or did they blurt my first and last name out for the other patients to hear?

Did I have to wait long, and if so was I informed of the delay immediately? Was a patient testimonial book, divided into surgical categories, available in the waiting room? Was the nurse friendly and interested in me as a person while she brought me to the consultation room, or was she monopolizing the conversation complaining about her recently deceased goldfish? Did I feel like another number heading for a conveyor belt to the operating room?

The office staff is an important part of any plastic surgeon's team. Ask your nonsurgical questions at the front desk. Questions such as when surgery will be scheduled or what time to arrive are matters for a patient coordinator. Most plastic surgeons have a coordinator on staff who manages these details, so the doctor can concentrate exclusively on you and your procedure.

## DOCTOR RADAR

On the flip side, it's amazing to me that some patients are rude to my front desk personnel or clinic nurse. The office staff alerts me if a patient is rude, angry, or overly demanding. Once a woman talked scathingly to my receptionist for several minutes in front of other patients, claiming she had gotten "poor directions" to the office. She received the same detailed, printed map all our patients receive. This is a patient who sends up red flags as a potentially unhappy customer. I knew I wouldn't operate on her after the way she had treated my staff. Luckily, she left without even seeing me.

## THE CONSULTATION

A nurse usually begins a consultation by taking the patient to an examination room and delivering some preliminary educational information, which often includes a video about the procedure you are interested in. When I enter the room, I introduce myself and usually make a joke about my long Polish last name. This not only breaks the ice, it gives me insight into how uptight a person is or if he or she has a sense of humor. I make small talk for a few minutes, reading the patient's responses. I conduct an exam to make sure the patient is a physically suitable candidate for the surgery they want, and discuss the procedure.

## A DOCTOR'S PERSPECTIVE

Once the exam-room portion of the visit is finished, I see prospective patients for a second time in my private office. I keep the shades closed during the consultation, so the person feels less distracted and safer, as if in a cocoon. To me, the metaphor of a cocoon is quite apt, because following surgery many patients do emerge with a new appearance. To add to the soothing environment, my office furniture is very comfortable, the same as you'd find in a living room. I use this atmosphere to put people at ease, so they can concentrate on the subject at hand and not be distracted by the view out the window, noise, or uncomfortable furniture.

I then give a little "surgery sermon" that explains the potential risks, limitations, and benefits of a procedure as it applies to the patient personally, and we talk about costs and any issues or questions the patient has. I look to see if people are reasonable and pleasant, if they're assertive or downright difficult. Occasionally, I meet with prospective patients who don't seem to grasp the limitations of plastic surgery or who are unsuitable candidates for it. If things go awry in the interview, I either refer patients to the colleague best qualified to handle their concerns or say that I'm uncomfortable with the interaction and explain why.

For example, one young man complained that everyone at his workplace was looking at his nose all the time. None of them liked him, he told me, because his nose was so large. He felt they were constantly laughing and talking behind his back. I noticed he had indicated on his health history that he had received treatment for a psychological condition. Further investigation with his therapist revealed a history of paranoid and delusional thinking. My surgery wouldn't have helped this man. I wrote a letter telling him this, and he never returned.

## A PATIENT'S POINT OF VIEW

You should be evaluating your potential surgeon in a similar way. Notice how you interact with the doctor. You want to be comfortable, but you also want someone who is technically excellent. Don't be swept off your feet by a suave and charming surgeon whose skills may not be outstanding. Plastic surgery is a high-ego business, so choose someone who isn't arrogant. Board-certified or not, there's a big difference between arrogance and confidence. If your surgeon can't remember your name, even with your chart in hand, how much personal attention do you think you are going to get?

On the other hand, personality isn't everything. I had a small procedure done on my face and went to the surgeon I considered the best in the world at this particular procedure. My focus was on skill, not bedside manner. But cosmetic procedures are very personal, and it is important to find a doctor you can communicate with openly and feel comfortable with. You have to weigh both skill and personality and find a surgeon you both like and trust.

One of my patients tells this story about interviewing doctors:

*"For years I had fantasized about having liposuction on my heavy thighs, but never really took the idea very seriously. Then a couple of things happened one summer. I unexpectedly came into some money that wasn't spoken for in my*

budget, and I was invited to go on a beach vacation in Mexico the following winter. So I decided to investigate a little further. I did some research, read a lot about the procedure on various websites, and got the names of a couple of doctors from my GP.

"The first one I saw, in a high-class suburban area, kept me waiting in a busy, grimy reception area for an hour after my scheduled appointment time. When I finally saw the doctor, who was clearly eager to finish up and go home, he seemed far more interested in what he thought I should look like than in finding out what I had in mind. When I asked about any risks involved with the procedure, his only response was to say that the biggest risk was that I would have unrealistic expectations and not be satisfied with the results because I didn't look like Christie Brinkley (who mentioned her??). In other words, if anything went wrong, it was my fault. That was it, and then it was off to see the office manager to discuss billing. Needless to say, I didn't have him perform my surgery.

"Next I had a consultation with Dr. Joe. The office was clean and calm, and I got in right on time. A nurse showed me a video about liposuction that discussed the risks as well as the benefits of the procedure. I had a pretty good idea of what they should be telling me from my own research, and they did a good job. They gave me a book of before and after photos and patient testimonials to look at. I had two meetings with Dr. Joe, one for an exam to make sure I was a good candidate and one to discuss the procedure. Everyone was very generous with time and information, even though it was a free consultation. Dr. Joe seemed interested in me as a person, not somebody he could try to mold into his own ideal fantasy woman. After that I didn't need to interview any more doctors. I had the procedure, and I'm delighted with the results."

**Dr. Joe's motto: When all else fails, listen to the patient.**

## CONSULTATION QUESTIONS

I try to be thorough and explain everything a patient needs to know about a procedure during our initial meetings, but I always leave plenty of time for questions. My advice is to be patient, sit tight, and produce your list of questions at the end of the interview to cover anything you aren't clear about. If a surgeon in any way scoffs at your questions, give your personal remodeling project to a kinder soul.

Don't be shy about asking questions, and don't be afraid of seeming nosy or suspicious. A reputable doctor will be happy to discuss his or her

## Overview of What to Ask at a Consultation

- Ask where the procedure will be performed.

- Ask about the doctor's hospital privileges.

- If the doctor operates a same-day surgery or office-based facility, ask if it's accredited.

- Ask who is ultimately responsible for your anesthesia – the surgeon or an anesthesiologist.

- Ask about the surgeon's experience in performing the procedure.

- Ask to see before and after photographs.

- Ask about the policy on surgical revisions.

- Ask what risks the procedure has in relation to your medical history.

- Ask what kind of result you can realistically expect.

- Ask what the expected recovery time is for your particular procedure.

qualifications. After all, it's your body, and this is real surgery. Here are some suggestions to get you started:

**Ask where the procedure will be performed.**

Cosmetic procedures can often be done either at private surgery centers or in hospitals. Usually, hospital prices are higher. Many same-day surgery facilities specialize in cosmetic surgery and offer competitive pricing. Most meet the highest standards of quality care. Be sure whatever facility your surgeon proposes to use is fully accredited.

One benefit of a private facility, compared to a hospital, is privacy. You may not want to have your name placed on a public surgical schedule at the local hospital where your neighbor works or your aunt volunteers. If you must have a procedure at the hospital, you can ask to use a pseudonym to keep your "nip and tuck" to yourself.

**Ask about a doctor's hospital privileges.**

Many surgical procedures can be safely performed in a doctor's office or other ambulatory surgical facility. Even so, find out if the doctor has operating privileges at an accredited hospital for the procedure you'd like to have. Before granting operating privileges, hospital credential committees evaluate a surgeon's training and competency for specific procedures.

I was chief of surgery at a major Twin Cities hospital, and I spent a year on the hospital's quality assurance committee and another year on its credential review committee. Not everybody applying for privileges at the hospital had appropriate training for the procedure they requested, and we turned them down. If the doctor doesn't have hospital privileges to perform your procedure, look for another surgeon. If you're uneasy with an answer regarding hospital privileges, call the hospital's medical affairs office. They should be able to answer your questions.

**If the doctor operates a same-day surgery or office-based facility, ask if it's accredited.**

If the operating room facility isn't accredited, be wary. Ask about the availability of life-saving equipment, the type of monitoring devices in the recovery area, and the facility's ancillary staff, which ideally should consist of registered nurses. Even though the facility might be perfectly safe, I wouldn't feel comfortable undergoing anesthesia unless the facility was fully accredited.

**Be sure to find out who administers anesthesia.**

**In my practice I always work with a board-certified anesthesiologist.** Some surgeons use nurse anesthetists rather than an MD anesthesiologist. Since I work with a board-certified anesthesiologist I'm free to be the artist doing my art project while the other doctor is taking care of you. **Be certain you know exactly who will be administering your anesthesia, what their credentials are, and who—the plastic surgeon or the anesthesiologist—is ultimately responsible for your anesthesia.**

**Ask about the surgeon's experience in performing the procedure.**

As a general rule, the more experience your surgeon has, the better your results are likely to be. Ask about a doctor's training, especially in new techniques. Ask to see training certificates, if you want more reassurance. Surgeons who are proud of their training have no problem displaying evidence of expertise. Ask how often the surgeon performs the procedure and with what success rate.

**Ask to see before and after photographs.**

I have a photo album filled with pre- and postoperative photographs of procedures I have performed. My practice's website also has many photographs. I never take offense at being asked about my experience in a certain area, and I am quick to back it up with concrete evidence. You can also ask for a list of patients who will talk to you about their experiences.

**Ask about the policy on surgical revisions.**

A small percentage of cases may require surgical revisions to achieve the desired results. Find out about any costs you'll have to pay. Many cosmetic surgeons don't charge a surgeon's fee for secondary or touch-up surgery within a reasonable time. Some surgeons, however, feel this encourages patients to seek frivolous additional surgery. This can be true in certain situations and I will, on rare occasion, charge a small fee as a disincentive to the patient who has extreme perfectionist tendencies. There may be a small fee for a surgical tray, and, when necessary, operating room and anesthesia charges.

Different types of surgery have different touch-up rates. Nationwide, about 15 percent of rhinoplasty patients seek revisions, for example. Even one of the top nasal surgeons in the country has a touch-up rate about equivalent to the national average (however, in many cases he is starting with difficult cases that already have had multiple surgeries). The bottom line is no matter who you see, there is always a chance that you will need a touch up.

In breast enlargement surgery, some implants migrate or deflate over the years. About one percent of breast implants fail each year. Ask if there is a replacement cost for the implant or additional operating room or surgeon's fees. The implant company I use provides a lifetime guarantee on the implant. For a limited period of time, they also cover facility fees including anesthesia, recovery room, and all supplies. Guarantees will vary, but I for one do not charge a surgeon's fee to replace an implant I've inserted within a certain period of time. However, if I'm redoing someone else's work, all fees apply.

**Ask what risks the procedure has in relation to your medical history.**

People with certain medical conditions, such as diabetes, may have a higher risk for certain complications with some procedures. For example, if you are a smoker, there are some procedures you shouldn't even consider. Heart problems or circulation disorders are among the other conditions that can affect your prognosis. Be sure to discuss your medical history honestly.

**Ask what kind of results you can realistically expect.**

If your stomach muscles have been weakened by a number of pregnancies, for example, liposuction alone may not be enough to give you a flat stomach again, and you might want to consider a tummy tuck. If you are willing to accept some remaining fullness, liposuction alone might be enough. Whatever the procedure, there will always be pros and cons that are influenced by your particular physique. Look for a surgeon who will discuss them honestly.

**Ask what the expected recovery time is for your particular procedure.**

Important points to discuss here are postoperative restrictions on activity and typical time periods for resuming work, family responsibilities, intimacy, and social activities.

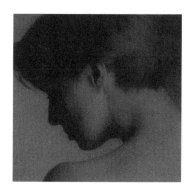

*chapter 4*

# HOW TO BE A TERRIFIC PATIENT, AND GET EVERYTHING YOU WANT FROM A PLASTIC SURGEON

"Remind yourself: This person will be changing

my body forever, and I'll look at it every day."

— Dr. John Tebbetts, Author of *The Best Breast*

*O*nce you've done your homework and found a doctor you're comfortable with, it's time to start thinking about the procedure itself. Keep in mind that just because you can do something doesn't mean that you should do it. Cosmetic surgery is a big step, and you should consider it very carefully. If it is the right thing for you, the results can be wonderful, but you have to do your part. This chapter will explain some of the details you need to know and give you some advice to help you get the surgery you want with the best possible results.

### ARE YOU SURE ENOUGH?

Choosing to change the way you look is a big decision. If I sense patients may be on the fence, I ask if they're 90 percent sure about the surgery. If they respond, "Yes, I'm 90 percent sure," I advise them not to have the procedure. I understand that people are anxious and nervous before having surgery. That's not what I'm talking about. I'm talking about a 100 percent commitment to having a procedure. If you are only 90 percent sure, that's a setup for trouble. In my experience, preoperative ambivalence directly correlates to postoperative dissatisfaction if anything goes wrong. A lack of up-front commitment can undermine a patient's resolve to weather the storm of a complication.

Plastic surgery is a blend of art and science. In this field, surgeons have preferences for surgical techniques. Choose a surgeon with whom you feel most comfortable and whose recommendations reflect your own best judgment. If you don't trust your surgeon, don't have the procedure. Don't be pressured for any reason whatsoever into a procedure you don't want or aren't ready to undergo.

### COMPUTER IMAGING AND PHOTOS

Many cosmetic surgeons employ computer imaging to help patients make up their minds about a procedure. A video camera or digital system takes your picture, and a split image is then projected onto a monitor so your photo appears on both sides of the screen. One of the preoperative images is modified to resemble what you would look like after surgery. Nose bumps can be removed, chin and neck profiles improved, subcutaneous fat recontoured, even breasts enlarged—quickly and painlessly. A hard copy can be printed for you.

But understand that this photo is not a guarantee of an exact outcome. Your surgeon may require you to sign a disclaimer that acknowledges this fact. One of the office assistants rather than the surgeon may do the imaging. Alternatively your doctor may use a marker to draw on a digital photograph to enhance your image. With your photo taken against a dark blue background, a blue pen or marker can be used to change a profile or contour to meet your wishes. Personally I prefer to draw on life-size photos, because I can calculate angles and balance proportions. These techniques are an excellent way to communicate your wish list and make sure you and your doctor are on the same wavelength.

## CONSULTATION DOS AND DON'TS

The results you get from your surgery can depend a lot on what kind of patient you are. It is vital to communicate honestly with your doctor about your needs and to be assertive about getting the procedure you want the way you want it. On the other hand, you have chosen your doctor because research assured he is a well-qualified professional, so it is equally important to respect your doctor's opinion and listen to recommendations. Here are some suggestions for getting the most out of your consultations with your doctors.

### Be specific.

For facial or body contouring surgery, I always ask patients to look in a mirror and describe what they want to change. They often try to pass the buck and ask me what I think. I tell them I'll put in my two cents after they have first related their concerns. The patient looks in the mirror and says "I don't like my nose," or "My nose is too big for my face," or "My nose is too long." The more specific you are, the better understanding a surgeon will have of your goals, and the better understanding you'll have of what's possible and what's not.

If you feel your nose is too long, for example, describe in which direction—either projecting too far from your face or extending too far down from the forehead, or possibly both. If you are uncomfortable with verbal description, ask to review pre- and postoperative photographs and point out what you like or dislike about them.

If you're having rhinoplasty or breast augmentation, bring in photos that show the results you'd like to see. This will help a surgeon better realize your dream.

On the other hand, make sure your dream is realistic. Don't bring in photos of models who are smiling yet have no facial wrinkles, for example. This doesn't represent reality. Photos of models are usually touched up and are often largely an illusion. If you expect to look like an airbrushed model after surgery, your surgeon will never be able to meet your expectations.

**Don't let your partner make decisions about your procedure.**

Sometimes a spouse or significant other accompanies a patient to the office. It's a very common situation with breast augmentation patients and sometimes with rhinoplasty and facelift patients. In one instance, a woman was explaining her goals while her husband was telling her how big he wanted her breasts to be. Often, the husband wants them larger than the patient does.

I had a breast augmentation patient return for a second visit with one of her female friends because she felt so pressured by her husband at the initial consultation. (To the men out there, be supportive, not pushy.) If you do bring a relative or friend to the office visit, advise that person to keep a low profile. Bring a supportive, caring person. This is the best companion to assist you with your important decisions.

**Give your doctor the benefit of the doubt.**

If your physician is late or hurried, come back for a second visit. Maybe it was just a very bad day. Everybody has them once in a while. I don't want to keep people waiting, but if I do, I often gain some valuable insights into how they handle "small stuff" stress. If they stay angry with me, imagine how hard it will be to nurse them through a complication. This may be enough for me to advise them to go elsewhere.

On the other hand, if you find yourself overreacting to things, maybe you are stressed about the idea of surgery and need to take a step back and reconsider. Maybe the timing is wrong for some reason. Pay attention to what you are telling yourself, and respect your instincts. You can always have the surgery at a later date, but you can't undo it once it is done.

**Don't interrupt.**

I go through a routine in my consultations, and if nervous patients or companions who want to control the situation continually interrupt, I might forget essential elements of the discussion. Occasionally, I have been interrupted to the point where I've forgotten to discuss something important with the patient. I've had to call them on the phone later to go through the missing information. Wait for your doctor to ask if you have any questions, then go over your list. If your potential surgeon is hard to understand, a poor communicator, or doesn't answer your questions, look elsewhere.

**Take no for an answer.**

A 71-year-old woman came to me who had been referred by her neighbor, on whom I had done a tummy tuck years before. This woman was unhappy with the fullness in her lower abdomen. She worked out regularly at a health club and did a lot of bicycling, weight lifting, and sit-ups. Nothing helped. So she decided she wanted liposuction.

Usually by age 70, skin tone is so poor that liposuction isn't beneficial without some type of skin lift along with the fat removal, but that doesn't necessarily rule out the procedure. In this case, however, the woman wasn't a candidate for other reasons. When I examined her, I discovered that she had very little subcutaneous fat in the belly area. Her protruding abdomen was actually caused by internal fat deposits that can't be removed with liposuction, combined with marked muscle relaxation.

We had a lengthy discussion, and I showed her a number of videos and photos. I explained that I didn't want to do a big surgery that wouldn't meet her expectations. Once she understood the limitations of the procedure, she thanked me for my honesty. I hope her understanding saved her from hunting around for a doctor who would tell her what she wanted to hear and perform the surgery, even if it wasn't likely to give her the results she wanted.

If someone still presses me in a situation like this, I almost always decline to perform the surgery. My advice is to accept it if your surgeon doesn't want to operate on you. You probably wouldn't be happy anyway. If you're still determined, you can always get a second opinion. Just be wary of searching until you finally find a surgeon who will act in his/her own best interests, not yours.

**Be scrupulously honest when filling out your medical history.**

Certain medical conditions can affect the surgical approach or anesthesia needs, and any prescription drugs you are taking will need to be taken into consideration. Even medications such as aspirin and other painkillers can thin the blood and can cause serious complications during surgery. During a breast enlargement, for example, a "dead space" is created where the implant is placed. If the patient is on one of these medications, their clotting abilities could be impaired and the space could fill with blood, causing complications.

Other substances that cause similar problems include more than 60 units of vitamin E per day, lecithin, garlic, fish oils, and shark cartilage supplements. Herbal medicines are biologically active and should be reported on your medical history. Echinacea, gingko, ginger, and other herbals will affect surgical procedures by either thinning the blood or changing the anesthetic requirements. St. John's Wort is an MAO inhibitor that affects the enzyme system for multiple physiological functions. Patients on an herbal MAO inhibitor such as this, even though it is mild, may experience a dramatic loss of blood pressure, a hypertensive crisis, or even death, depending on which medications were used.

Many years ago, one of my patients developed a horrific bleeding complication during a facelift. She had undergone other medical surgeries in the past without bleeding problems, but this time the bleeding was so severe it required many additional hours in the operating room. The patient also had to return for a second procedure the following day to drain collected blood, called a hematoma, in the facial area. Upon further questioning, the patient revealed she had been taking large amounts of lecithin daily. Lecithin has been used to help prevent heart attacks and strokes because it thins the blood.

I give all of my patients a card describing most of these blood-thinning or potentially life-threatening medications and herbals that should be reported and avoided for two weeks before and after surgery.

## Consultation Overview

- Don't dress up or down for the consultation. Be yourself.

- Bring a list of questions and photos you've gathered.

- Enter the consultation process with a friendly attitude and an open mind.

- Be patient if the doctor is late.

- Save your questions until the end. Most will be answered during the course of your consultation.

- Bring a notepad and take notes. Studies show that the average patient retains only 35 percent of what was discussed after 24 hours.

- Realize that you may have selective hearing about the downside of the procedure.

- If you're sure about having the procedure, get a written estimate of the fee.

**Don't lie about nicotine use.**

It could seriously jeopardize your outcome. I have an information card that explains the dangers of nicotine and second-hand smoke, and even Nicorette gum and nicotine patches. Every time nicotine enters the body, blood vessels go into spasm, limiting blood flow, which can jeopardize a new surgical area. Nicotine use should be further discussed with your physician. Discontinuing smoking is recommended for all surgeries but is essential in some, like abdominoplasties and facelifts.

I've seen two dramatic complications with patients who were less than honest about nicotine use. In the first, a breast reduction patient's left nipple turned stone-cold blue the night after surgery. There were no pressure dressings in the breast, and no discernible reason for the problem. I applied a vasodilator to help open up the blood vessels in the breast and throughout her body. What I didn't know was that she had been sneaking out of the hospital to smoke. Because of her smoking, a portion of the nipple died, and I had to graft skin and reconstruct the lost areas. Despite reading the information on smoking, she still had been puffing away.

In the second case, the patient suffered skin loss—where the skin dies and sloughs off—after a facelift. This complication was completely unexplainable. Before surgery, this patient stated she didn't smoke, the major cause of postoperative skin loss. She was given our smoking information card and throughout the weeks of recovery repeatedly denied any contact with nicotine, either directly or indirectly. In fact, she asserted she had never smoked in her life.

I felt terrible about this complication that seemingly had no cause. I even flew to Dallas to learn a completely new facelift procedure from an innovative and pioneering surgeon that was supposed to alleviate the risk of skin loss. Several weeks later, at a restaurant for our office Christmas party, my office manager suddenly nudged me in the ribs. "Look who's at the table next to us," she said. Sure enough, our facelift patient, the woman who had never smoked, was sitting there chain smoking, and my belief in the law of cause and effect was reestablished.

Many surgeons, including myself, won't perform a facelift on patients who smoke. Possibly as a result, research indicates that many patients who claim to have recently stopped smoking are not telling the truth. As unfair as it may seem, we have to assume that patients might not stop smoking and will experience skin loss from a procedure. I try to take patients' statements at face value and believe it if they say they will quit. We even shake on it, but I know in the back of my mind they might be cheating.

The moral of these stories is that your surgeon, I hope, is your professional friend. Don't turn it into an adversarial relationship by withholding pertinent information. You could do yourself some serious harm.

## SURGICAL COMPLICATIONS

Over 11 million cosmetic surgical procedures are performed annually, ASAPS statistics show. Consumer demand for cosmetic surgery is increasing steadily. Public concern about the safety of cosmetic surgery is also rising. What about the disasters we read about in the newspapers? How can a person possibly die from a simple cosmetic procedure? After all, isn't this just "surface surgery?" Do patients die from plastic surgery because doctors don't know what they're doing, or is it just bad luck or a rare allergic reaction?

The chance of an anesthesia allergy is less than one in a million, so death under that circumstance is rare. The chance of a healthy patient dying in an auto accident driving to the operation is greater than the chance of dying from the surgery. Most cases of surgical death involved a prolonged procedure that often included administering massive amounts of fluid to replace volume lost.

I recently read a newspaper article about problems with an extremely long procedure, lasting some 13 hours. The length of the surgery might not be the direct cause of death but could be a contributing factor. I try to limit surgery to less than five hours. High-volume liposuction—removing more than about five liters of subcutaneous tissue, equivalent to eleven pounds—puts a patient at higher risk for fluid shifts, fluid overload, blood clots, or fat clots. I generally limit suction lipectomy volumes to eleven pounds or less, and if additional volume is removed, the procedure is done in a hospital.

In one reported death from liposuction, allegedly unsterilized equipment was the culprit. This was simply poor medicine in a small practitioner's office (not a plastic surgeon) where the sterilization equipment wasn't working properly. You can help avoid complications like this by checking to be sure that the procedure will be performed in an accredited facility.

In another reported case, a patient died from a surgical infection after the bowel was perforated during liposuction surgery. This is a rare case, but surgery does carry risks, and the only way not to have a complication is not to operate.

The cards can be stacked in your favor, however, by seeking an appropriately trained practitioner. Plastic surgeons have basic training in the treatment of shock, blood loss, fluid and electrolyte shifts, fluid overload, and anesthesia complications. Only practitioners with this extensive background should perform procedures such as liposuction, and particularly high-volume liposuction. They have the appropriate training to manage a patient and handle any complications.

The percentage of complications in cosmetic procedures is very low as long as the following safeguards are in place:
- The case is not prolonged.
- An excessive volume is not being removed.
- The medical facility is accredited.
- The surgeon uses appropriate sterile techniques.
- The surgeon has performed appropriate preoperative analysis, physical examination, and technical execution of the procedure.
- The patient complies with preoperative precautions.
- The patient is completely truthful and forthcoming about their medical history.

## PAY IN ADVANCE? YOU'VE GOT TO BE KIDDING!

Now we get to the burning question for many patients: How much will surgery cost? Insurance doesn't cover cosmetic surgery. Advance payment is usually required and is common practice nationally. The good news is that cosmetic surgery fees haven't been increasing as fast as the cost of living. In fact, the cost of plastic surgery hasn't risen as fast as the price of other "optional" purchases such as a new car.

Most plastic surgery patients come from households with average incomes. Many of my patients have saved for years to pay for their surgical procedures. Patients must compare the costs with the benefits. Plastic surgery is an investment in self-esteem. For people who are so bothered by their appearance that it affects their enjoyment of life and their perception of themselves, the cost of plastic surgery is money well spent.

The American Society of Plastic Surgeons endorses a financing program for patients. Market research showed that many people who wanted plastic surgery delayed a decision because they couldn't pay in advance. The society's program gives candidates for plastic surgery a chance to pay for their care slowly, over time. This financing program has worked well for many patients in my office. You might inquire about it during your fact-finding process.

Also, costs of plastic surgery vary depending on the patient's needs. For example, liposuction will vary from one patient to another in terms of volume and the number of areas treated. Cosmetic surgery overall is a very personalized service, and fees will relate to the extent of the procedures done and the level of difficulty. Fees also vary in different parts of the country and among surgeons.

Sometimes when I ask for payment in advance, patients complain that I don't trust them. Most patients are reliable about money, but some aren't. I explain that it's our office policy to have all patients pay two weeks prior to surgery. I can't deviate from that policy by singling out a certain patient to favor. I explain I have every reason to trust them but to have surgery they must comply with office guidelines and rules.

The pay-in-advance policy is followed nationwide, and for very good reason. Studies show that patients who don't pay in advance of cosmetic surgery tend to find an incredible number of defects in the surgical outcome. Large percentages go on to withhold payment based on real or fictitious complaints. After all, cosmetic surgery isn't like buying a new car—nobody will make you give it back if you claim you aren't happy with it.

Some surgeons discuss money directly with their patients, and some don't. A surgery coordinator might go over fees. Be sure to obtain fees in writing. I provide a copy of a surgical cost estimate, which gives details and cost of each procedure to be performed. The patient then initials and dates the fee quote and receives a copy. This helps avoid misunderstandings that often arise when money and medicine mix.

Costs include the surgeon's fee and fees for the surgical facility and anesthesia. Other

## Notes on Cost and Payment

- Financing for cosmetic procedures may be available from the American Society of Plastic Surgeons.

- Fees will vary depending upon the extent of the procedure, the level of difficulty, as well as the geographical location of the surgeon.

- The pay-in-advance policy is followed nationwide and is meant to protect the surgeon from false complaints. Studies show that patients who don't pay in advance tend to find an incredible number of defects in the surgical outcome.

- Be sure to obtain a list of fees in writing.

- Remember that the cost of a procedure will include surgeon's fees, fees from the surgical facility and the cost of anesthesia. In many cases you will be asked to pay the surgeon and the surgery center separately.

possible costs are the preoperative physical and blood work, pathology reports, postoperative medications, surgical garments, and private-duty nursing. Patients write one check to me and one to a surgery center. When possible, I do the preoperative physical examination to save patients money. Private-duty nursing is available, but at an additional cost. It's less expensive to have a family member help you following the procedure.

## SOME WORDS ABOUT INSURANCE COVERAGE

Some surgical procedures are a combination of cosmetic and reconstructive surgery, which is often covered by insurance. The insurance reimbursement will vary based on your policy, but fees for the reconstructive portion of a surgery ethically can't be increased to cover any portion of a cosmetic procedure, and insurance companies have "reasonable and customary fees" on which they base payments. For example, nasal surgery is often a combination of cosmetic surgery and surgery for breathing problems. Cosmetic work is an out-of-pocket expense, and breathing and reconstructive work is billed to insurance.

For the rare insurance cases I do, I usually write a letter for prior authorization, so the insurance company will provide some assurance that they will subsequently cover the procedure's cost. This gives patients peace of mind, and in many cases is mandatory to obtain coverage. Some flexible health care reimbursement plans allow deposits that can be used for cosmetic surgery. In my experience, most don't. Review the rules of your employer's plan or consult your employer's benefits professional. And as a side note, cosmetic surgery is not tax deductible, although you might want to check with your tax adviser to be sure.

Even though most cosmetic procedures aren't covered by insurance, some people keep on trying. One morning I received a letter from the husband of a liposuction patient. He wrote that to obtain flex-plan monies, I had to write his company a letter stating the surgery was medically necessary. What was I supposed to tell them, that his wife had an acute fat attack? Please don't ask your doctor to lie for you. It is dishonest and unethical. And think about it—do you really want to trust your surgery to a doctor who is willing to lie to an insurance company to get your business? It doesn't exactly inspire confidence.

Insurance does pay for medically necessary procedures, but that can become complicated as well. Paperwork is escalating, especially since the advent of managed care. Health insurance companies used to trust doctors to make appropriate surgical judgments, but now most procedures are questioned and must be authorized in advance. Sometimes appeal letters need to be written, compounding the amount of time spent on a situation that would have been on autopilot twenty years ago.

I tell my office staff if they can't find me to look under my paperwork. Sometimes it feels like I'm being buried in it. Paperwork is costly in time and money. Even though I now limit my practice to cosmetic procedures, most of which don't involve insurance, it takes forever to clear my desk before I go home. When I return from a two-week stint doing surgeries in South America, several foot-high piles of paperwork sit on my desk. But it's part and parcel of the job and must be done.

The bottom line is that insurance companies will pay for medically necessary procedures, but you and your doctor will probably have to jump through some paperwork hoops first. If you think your procedure might be covered, discuss it with your surgeon.

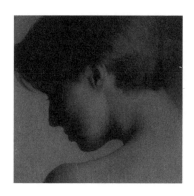

*chapter 5*

# DOCTOR AND PATIENT
# RELATIONSHIPS

"If your preoperative evaluation suggests that your

patient is emotionally or psychologically at risk,

trust your judgement; good judgement

usually comes from bad experiences."

— Dr. Rod J. Rohrich, MD
Past President of The American Society of Plastic Surgeons (ASPS) and
Editor-in-Chief, *Plastic and Reconstructive Surgery Journal*

*I*t's common for patients to feel close to their surgeons. You wouldn't be the first person to develop some affection for your doctor. In reality, as a patient you don't know your physician as a person. It's the "magic" the surgeon performs—not the person—that's the draw. To take the relationship with your doctor outside the clinical setting isn't fair to either of you.

These are boundary issues. When we cross boundaries our roles become blurred, which can lead to misunderstanding. I wear different hats in different situations. If I'm operating on a close colleague, I'm surgeon first, colleague second. If my friend mixes up these hats and merges our roles, I might not do the surgery.

If I run into a patient at a social engagement, I'm careful not to acknowledge the person. This could breach doctor-patient confidentiality. One of two things usually happens: The patient either moves away from me or interacts with me on a purely social level, as if we've never met. Less frequently, a patient touts my services. A large part of my practice is composed of friends referred by prior patients. I consider this as the highest possible compliment and tell patients so in a thank-you letter.

## DEPENDENCY NEEDS

Many patients become dependent and needy, especially if they have a complication. You must ride out the situation together. The surgeon certainly has no choice, although the patient can choose to go elsewhere. That's why it's so important to sort out in the initial consultation whether this is the surgeon for you and, from my perspective, whether this is the patient for me. Can I weather a storm with this person?

Some cosmetic surgery patients become angry and depressed if things don't go perfectly, and they let me know about it. I feel badly when they say, "If I had known this was going to happen, I never would have had the surgery." At the same time, I'm thinking, "If I had known this was going to happen, I never would have done the surgery on you." Some patients have decent results but still focus on the slightest imperfections. The patient who does this may have a dependent personality and need longer office visits and more attention overall.

## THE NARCISSIST

Another personality type that doesn't do well with an unexpected outcome, or even a good one, is the narcissistic patient, who usually comes in for multiple consultations prior to surgery. This type of patient also may be somewhat hostile and suspicious of the physician. The narcissist expects perfection and invariably thinks the outcome didn't meet expectations.

## THE GIFT-BEARER

Just about all the plastic surgeons I know receive gifts from grateful patients. In general, these are sincere, appreciative expressions of gratitude. Occasionally, I'm put on guard by patients bringing gifts because they expect reciprocity. Perhaps they want more surgery, and they're fishing for a discount. Usually they slip from calling me "Dr. Joe" to simply "Joe." They change the conversation from surgery to whether I'm staying in shape or what plans I have for the weekend. These subtle changes put me on guard to stay in the proper role. If you want to show your appreciation, think about a gift of flowers to the entire staff or a donation to a charity in your doctor's name.

## THE JUNKIE

A while back, a talk show featured a woman who underwent dozens of surgical procedures because she wanted to look like Barbie. Perhaps it's the illusion of looking like a fantasy figure, or an attempt to undo the past, satisfy a deep need to change, or just look younger, but some patients keep coming back for more. I would say most of my repeat patients are somewhat driven, but generally have a healthy desire to simply improve their appearance. I don't see them as neurotic but as satisfied clients returning for more. On some afternoons my entire consultation schedule is with previous patients. I take this as a compliment.

If I do feel a patient is overdoing it, I tell them so. I've seen plastic surgery junkies who have fallen out of favor with their previous surgeons. I've found these patients usually aren't good candidates for further surgery, and I try to persuade them not to proceed. I might even tell them I'm feeling a little uncomfortable and suggest noninvasive ways to enhance their appearance such as skin care, vein removal, collagen, *The Zone Diet*, exercise, or a personal trainer. Sometimes saying no is the best way to help an individual.

## DEALING WITH COMPLAINTS

In my practice, the complaint window is always open. If patients do complain, I believe that my role is to remain calm and supportive. Instead of resisting complaining patients, I now look at them as trying to help me. After all, they're a self-selected subgroup of perfectionists. Complainers point out flaws, and this helps me to become a better surgeon. Instead of becoming defensive, I listen to exactly what they have to say. I look for what is true to me, and don't take it personally. Many patients, I've learned, just want to be heard. They don't want me to put on my Mr. Fix-It hat.

Sometimes, patients don't want to hurt my feelings, so they complain to a nurse. I've asked my staff to alert me when this happens, so the problem can be addressed immediately. Some issues are legitimate, and we do everything we can to take care of the problem. It's important to give feedback to your surgeon, even if it's negative. Of course, we also like to hear about what went right.

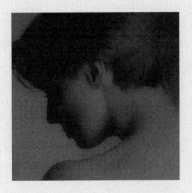

# Part 2 : Procedures

This section describes a variety of cosmetic procedures, with information about the surgery, its risks and complications, recovery period, and general costs. If you're having a procedure done, you will receive preoperative and post-operative instructions from your doctor with more details about the specific requirements for your surgery. Please use your doctor's instructions as your primary guidelines and follow them carefully. The information provided here is more general and will give you a good overview of the various procedures available, but it shouldn't replace your doctor's recommendations.

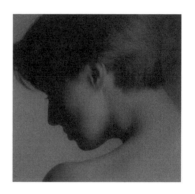

*chapter 6*

# BREAST SURGERIES

"Breast surgery is a very sensitive, personal,
and individual decision. What could be more radical
than actually changing the body part many women
connect most directly with their femininity?"

– Anonymous

## BREAST AUGMENTATION

Breast augmentation is a popular surgery among women. It certainly is my most common surgery. Nationally, the average age of a woman seeking this procedure is around 32. **However my patients range from age 18 to women in their 60s.** The average patient likely has had two or more children and has breast-fed at least one of them. Breast-feeding can cause the skin and breast tissue to lose elasticity. This causes breasts to sag and sometimes involute, which means they actually become smaller. In fact most women's breasts become smaller after bearing children even if they don't breast-feed.

*"My breasts were always small, but I never wanted them to be surgically altered until after my baby was born,"* one patient wrote. *"They turned into nothing. I take care of myself by eating well and exercising. Having my chest look like a little boy's chest really bothered me."*

Breast augmentation can:

- Enhance breast size or shape.
- Restore breast volume or shape lost through pregnancy. This isn't vanity. Many women are simply reclaiming their past figures from B.C. (Before Children).
- Help your clothes and swimwear fit better.
- Correct asymmetries or differences in breast size.
- Reconstruct breasts after mastectomy for cancer or premalignant conditions.

*"By having a breast augmentation you are not trying to change your body, you are enhancing what is already beautiful,"* wrote one of my patients.

An interesting study was done among women who underwent breast implantation. Initially, many of the women were shocked by the change and felt they had made a terrible mistake because their breasts were too large. Six months after surgery, 90 percent of the women said they were okay with the size. One year later, 90 percent wished the implants were larger. So I counsel my patients that one year after the operation, there is a 90 percent chance they will wish they had had bigger implants.

*"Before my surgery, I had this huge fear of ending up with enormous breasts and of looking very fake,"* one patient wrote. *"I trusted Dr. Joe and agreed with his advice to go to a bigger size. My end result is wonderful."*

**Waking up in the recovery room and seeing their new breasts for the first time is one of the most exciting parts of the surgery. However many women feel they have two huge, hard torpedoes glued to their chest, instead of natural soft breasts. The implants may be swollen for a few days, and are naturally tight. Their new breasts will soften gradually and take on a more natural shape over the next six months.**

Many patients also are reluctant to go as big as they want because of worries the change will be too obvious. I tell them to go home, start stuffing their bras with silk stockings or handkerchiefs, and wear loose clothing. That way the change won't be as noticeable. If a patient suddenly appears larger overnight, an acutely aware person (usually her mother!) may put it all together.

So how do you decide which size to pick? Terms like "bigger," "not too big," and "just enough," don't communicate your image too clearly. "Big to you and big to me are two different things," I tell my patients. Placing implants of various sizes or plastic bags filled with rice into your bra may be slightly more helpful. I measure a patient's rib cage, breast fold, tissue thickness, breast width, and even the distance to the belly button and shoulders during my examination to better ascertain how she will carry a certain size implant. Careful measuring helps me to better appreciate what she and God are giving me to fashion. They say a picture is worth a thousand words. In the case of breast augmentation, it's worth 10 times more. I sometimes ask patients to bring in pictures from Victoria's Secret or a similar catalog to help me understand what breast size they want. They can also choose from our office preop and postop photo album. One to three pictures is sufficient because any more can be confusing. **I refer frequently to these pictures in the operating room as I perform the procedure.**

*"Goodbye girls, hello ladies,"* exclaimed one patient as she drifted off to sleep in the operating room.

Once the implants are inserted, I sit the patient up while she is still asleep. Then I walk around and look at my work from every angle, constantly adjusting the implants' position and size. I try my best as an artist and a human being to match the pictures she has brought in. I tell patients, "I'm an artist, but I'm also trying to be a mind reader." I want to give each woman what she envisions, and pictures help me do that.

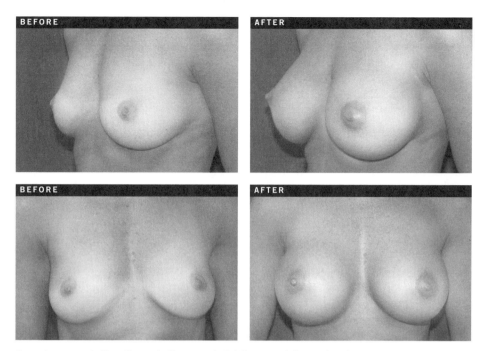

Breast augmentation through the armpit (oblique and front views)

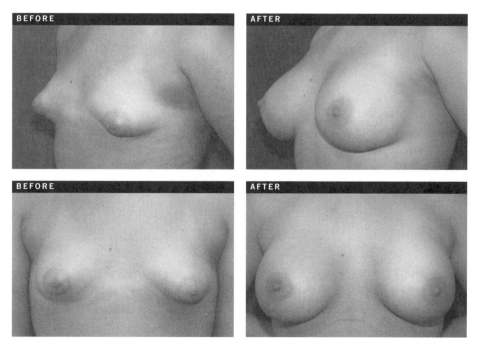

Breast augmentation and correction of developmental asymmetry
(oblique and front views)

I also encourage patients to review my website, **www.tcplasticsurgery.com**. You can look for patients with your body proportions, age, height, weight and cup size both preop and post op. Pay attention to any differences you may see in the preop photos from one side to the other. You can print these out and bring them in as well. Rank your photos in terms of size and implant position—just right, a little too high, too low, whatever—and write your notes on the picture. Be frank about your expectations. Too many pictures—more than two or three—can be confusing, however.

Many patients want cleavage from breast enlargement, but often this is not possible. I release the muscle attachments as far toward the middle of the breastbone as I can, but after that it's between you and God (or a really great bra) whether or not you will have cleavage. If you have a wide space between your breasts because of a broad sternum, you will never have cleavage.

### Implant Types

I use both silicone and saline implants. Silicone gel implants look more natural and feel softer with less chance of visible wrinkling. Studies show silicone implants do not increase the incidence of disease or the chances of developing breast or other cancers. The FDA recommends MRI scans to follow gel implants postop. Saline implants, on the other hand, are less expensive. I can insert a saline implant through a smaller incision and can more easily adjust for minor size discrepancies between each breast during surgery. Implants come in various shapes. About 99 percent of the time, I insert a standard round implant. Discuss the pros and cons of each shape with your surgeon.

### The Procedure

I favor putting implants under the chest muscle because my radiology colleagues think this position interferes less with mammography and the early detection of breast cancer than if the implant is placed on top of the muscle. Not all surgeons agree on this, but I like to err on the side of caution. The alternative is to place the implant on top of the muscle but under the breast tissue. The incidence of irregularities is much higher when the implant is placed on top of the muscle in a patient who has little overlying breast tissue to cover the edges of a saline implant (incidentally, this isn't as big a problem with silicone).

Potential approaches to insertion include incisions in the armpit, around the areola, in the crease at the base of the breast, or even through the belly button. **I let the woman decide on the location of her incision.** Most women choose the armpit incision because they don't want a cut on their breasts.

The incision is the entry point I will use to create a pocket for an implant. Once the implant is in position, the incision is closed.

Before we begin surgery I use a marker to draw the incisions and the entire surgical plan on a patient's chest. I guess the body is the ultimate canvas on which to draw. The plan includes the type of incision (the patient picks one of three incisions), implant size on each side (equal amounts on each side or more on one side if the breast is smaller), placement of the implant (high, middle or low) and finally placement toward the inside or outside of the breastbone. While looking in a mirror she verifies our plan is exactly what she has in mind. Crystal-clear communication is essential to ensure the patient gets the results she wants.

Patients take three *Hibiclens (chlorhexidene)* showers the night before surgery. Washing the chest and armpits helps prevent infection. During surgery I give a specific intravenous antibiotic which kills the exact germ implicated in the formation of breast implant capsules (firmness). Surgery is done on a same-day basis and takes less than 30 minutes to complete. With modern techniques, many patients have surgery on a Friday and are back to work on Monday. Pain medication is prescribed to alleviate any discomfort. I also prescribe a muscle relaxer and anti-nausea medication. Patients may not have to take antibiotic pills after surgery.

*"I wasn't really in that much pain,"* one patient wrote. *"I just felt really stiff and tight. Most of the pain I did have was easily controlled by my medications."*

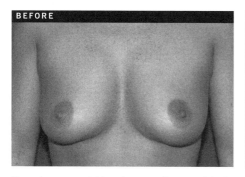
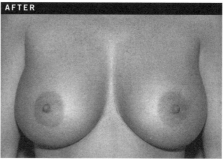

Breast augmentation for a patient reclaiming her pre-pregnancy figure

*"I was tired of going to the gym and looking like the guy on the machine next to me. Now I look and feel like a woman,"* said one of my patients.

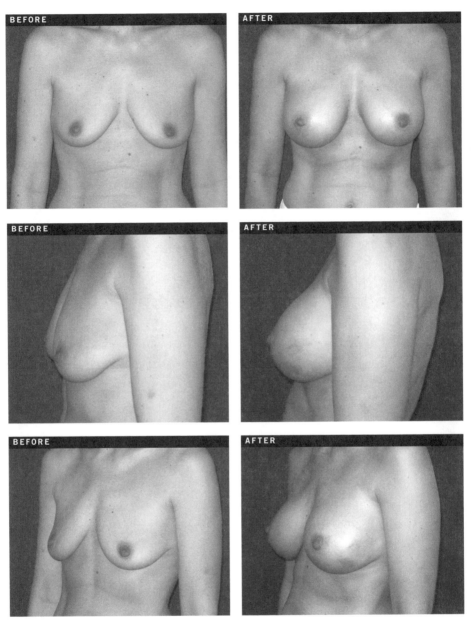

Silicone gel implants placed through the armpits to enhance breast volume and shape after pregnancy

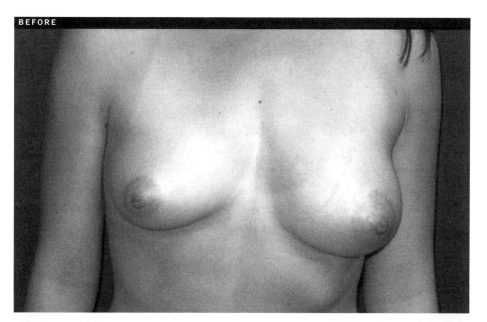

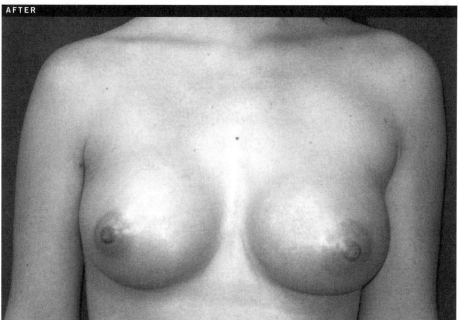

Incomplete development of the right breast in a 19-year-old patient, corrected with bilateral breast augmentation

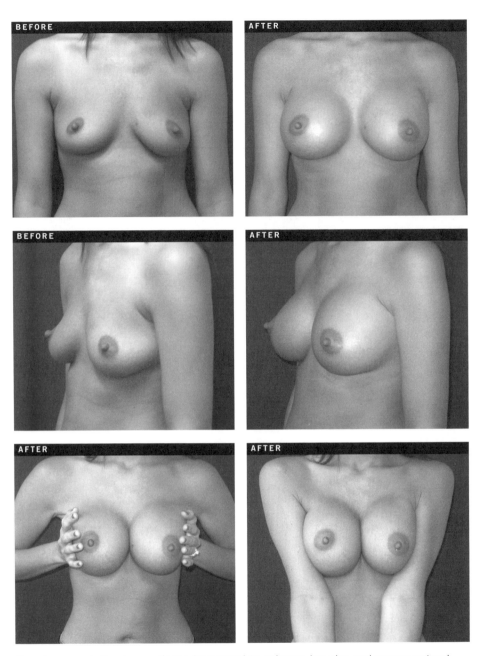

Breast augmentation in a patient who wanted to enhance her size and appear natural.
Note the softness of her implants.

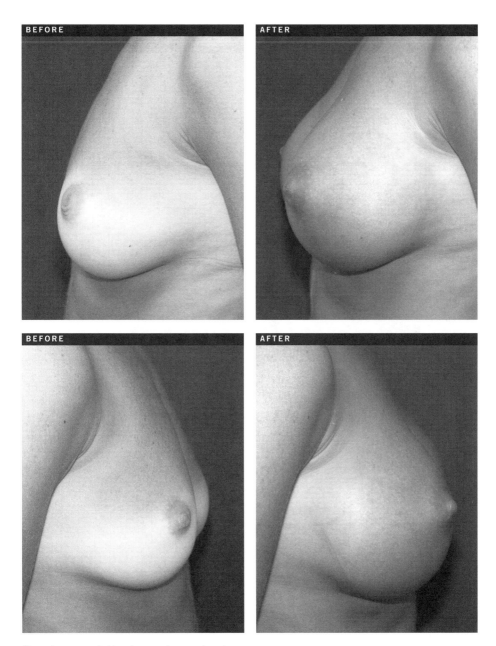

Breast augmentation to create a natural appearance

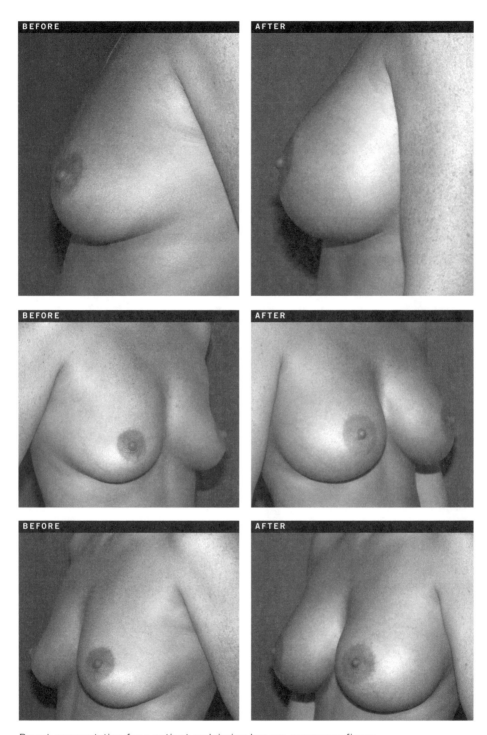

Breast augmentation for a patient reclaiming her pre-pregnancy figure

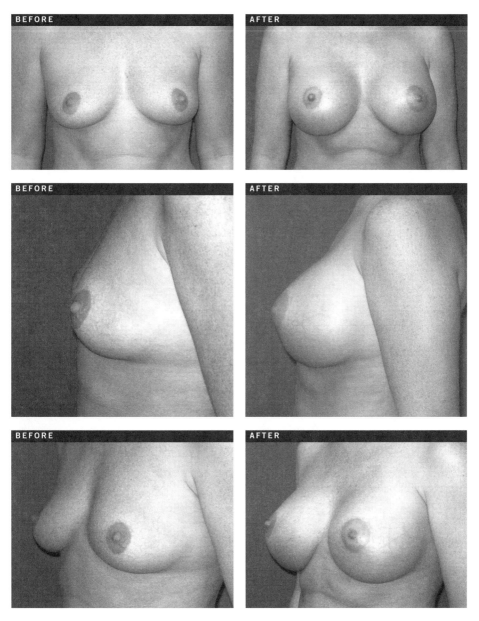

This patient requested breast augmentation to give "body" to her breasts.

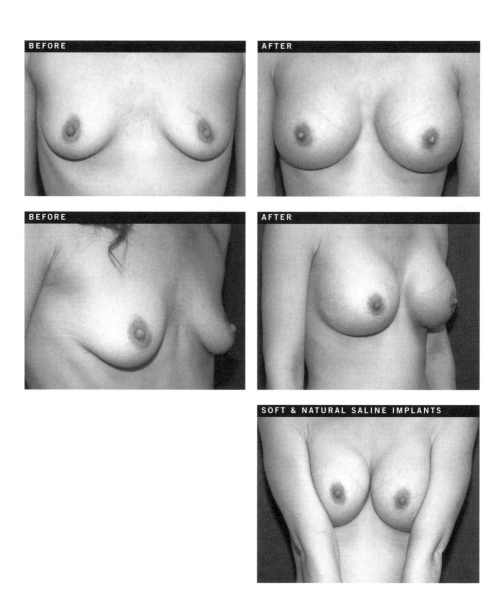

This patient wanted to regain her figure from "B.C." (Before Children). Note the softness of her implants.

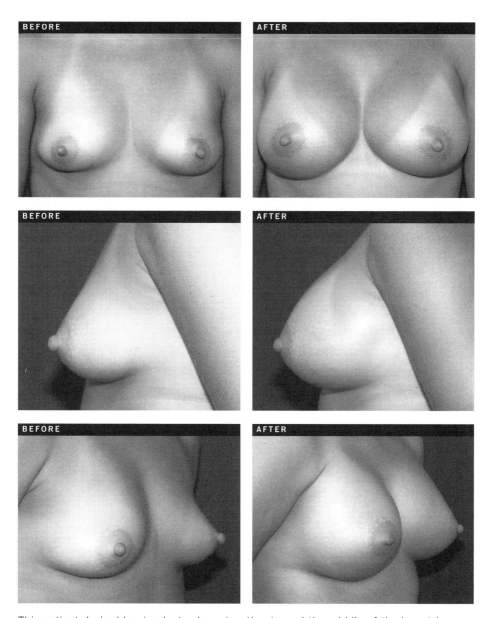

This patient desired her implants closer together toward the middle of the breast bone.

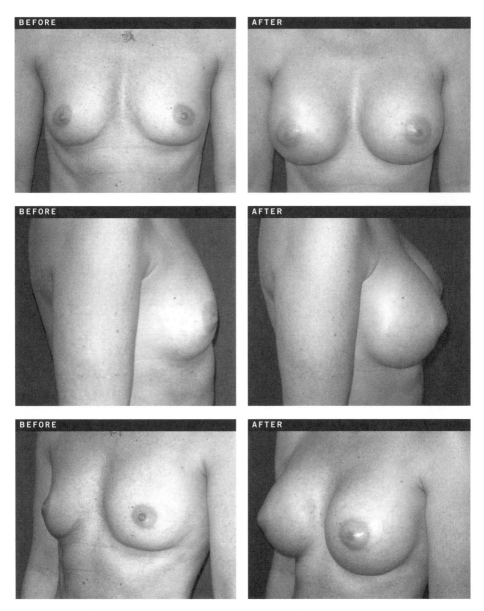

Breast augmentation centered on the nipple (multiple views)

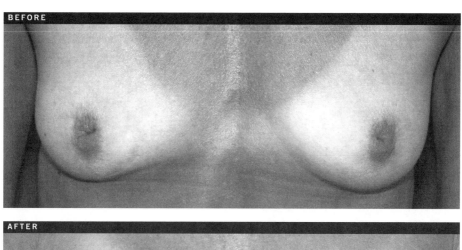

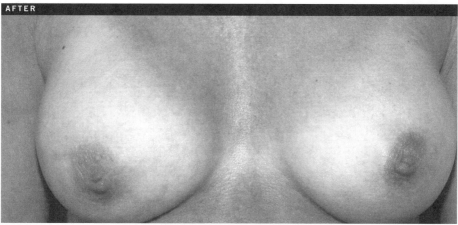

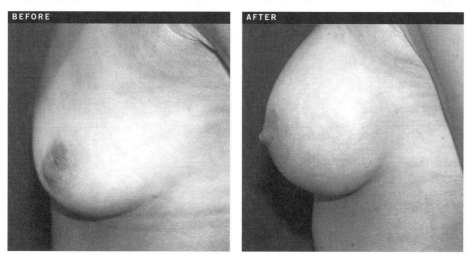

Occasionally breast augmentation will help inverted nipples. This patient suffered from inverted nipples which were corrected by breast augmentation with smooth, round saline implants placed under the chest muscle.

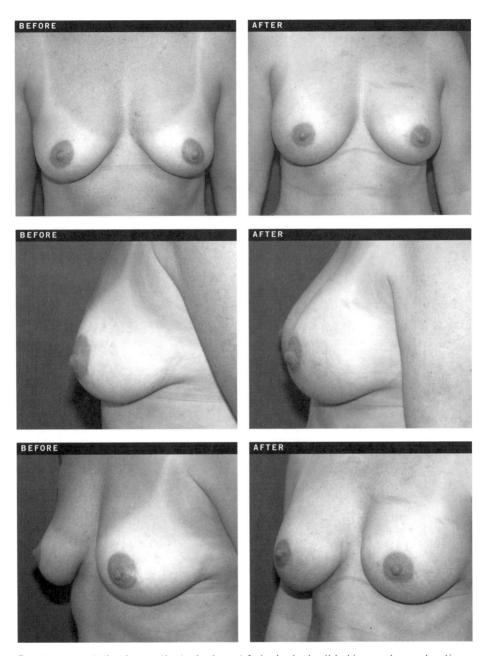

Breast augmentation in a patient who breast-fed: she had mild skin envelope relaxation with good nipple height above the breast fold

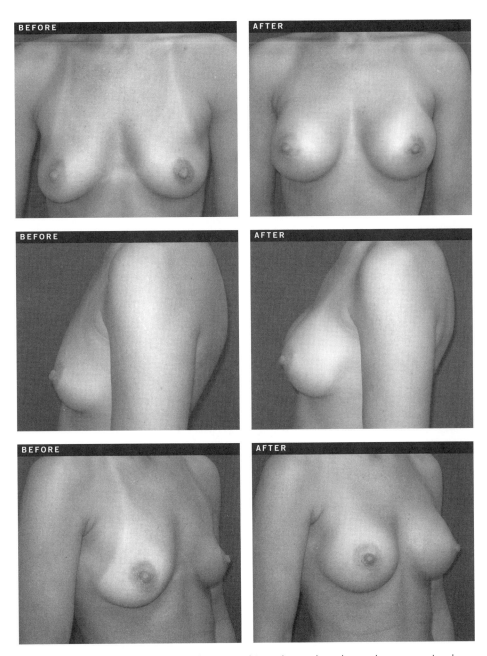

Breast augmentation in a patient who wanted to enhance her size and appear natural

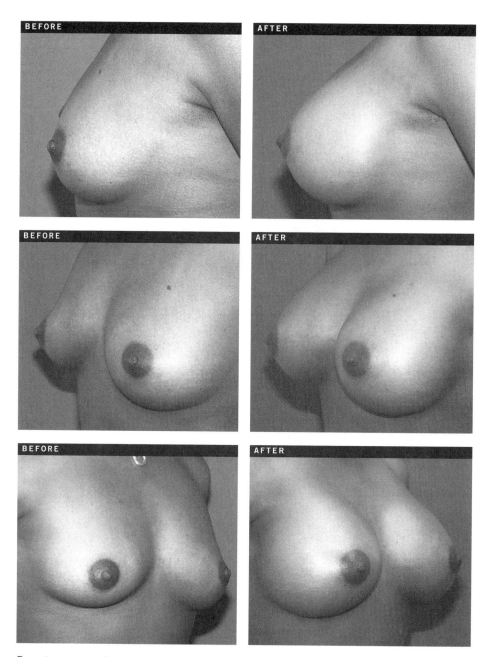

Breast augmentation through the armpit

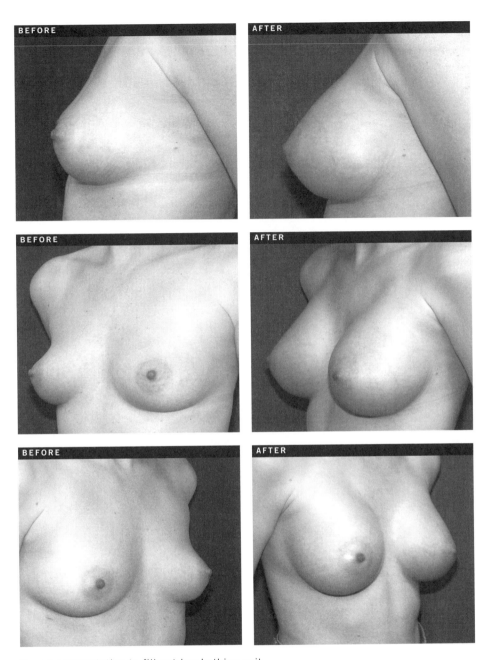

Breast augmentation to fill out her bathing suit

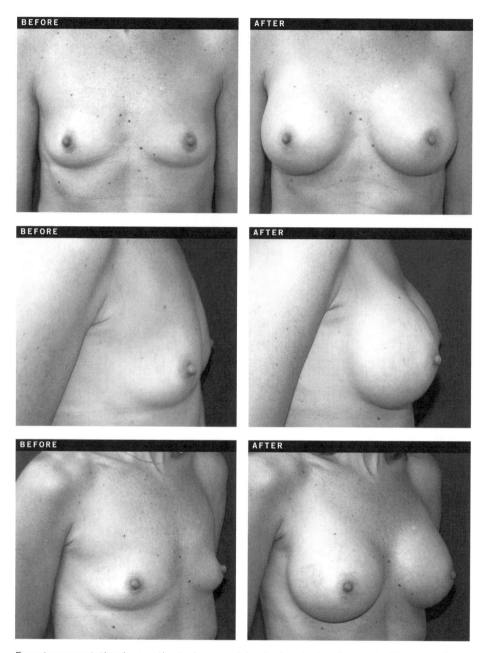

Breast augmentation in a patient who complained of underdevelopment of her breasts

## DUAL-PLANE AUGMENTATION

Seventeen percent of my augmentations are done with a dual-plane approach to lift breast tissue, elevate the nipple-areolar complex, and release a tight breast crease. This is technically a breast enlargement procedure—I call it the "internal lift." It creates a breast pocket above and below the muscle (hence the term "dual") where an implant is inserted. By releasing the breast attachments on top of the muscle, the breast slides upward around the implant. This technique avoids the more extensive scars of an external lift, and can be especially useful in fixing early sagging.

## RAPID RECOVERY BREAST AUGMENTATION

I specialize in rapid recovery breast augmentation, also known as the "no-touch technique," a surgical procedure that uses special instruments and techniques to minimize tissue damage and avoid touching the ribs (hence the term "no-touch"). It causes far less trauma to the surrounding tissue than traditional approaches and dramatically reduces my patients' pain and suffering as well as their recovery time. After I began using this technique, my staff and I interviewed each patient postoperatively to assess the results. We discovered 95 percent returned to normal daily activities within 24 hours. (For more information, see Dr. John Tebbetts' book, *The Best Breast*, CosmetXpertise, 1999.)

Before I began using the rapid recovery method, a substantial number of my patients would spend as much as two to three weeks stiffened with pain. Now I have a patient who reported that she had folded three loads of laundry and bathed her two boys the evening after surgery. A second patient worked a full day at her office the day after her surgery. Another went to a movie eight hours postoperatively.

The patient shown doing arm exercises and smiling less than 24 hours postoperatively was one of my first patients to use the no-touch technique. She was off all prescription analgesics the day after surgery and drove herself to the office for her follow-up exam. This is not magic, but it sometimes seems that way compared to the old methods. My staff and I, as well as the anesthesiologists and recovery room nurses, absolutely, unequivocally see a significant difference in my patients' recovery times. I now recommend this technique for almost all of my breast augmentation patients.

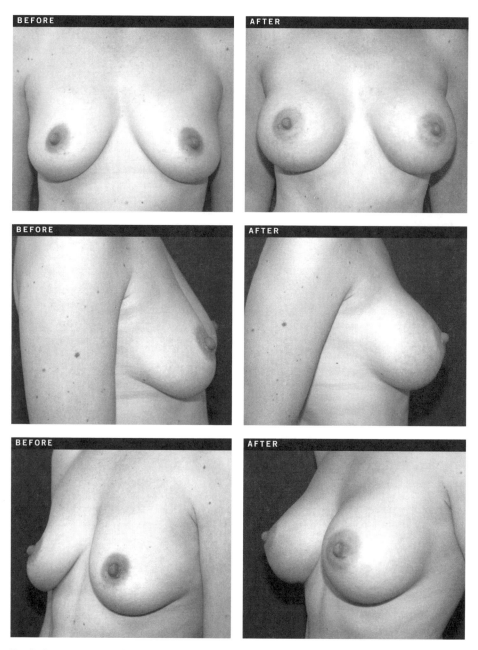

Dual-plane augmentation: limited incision "internal breast lift" for laxity

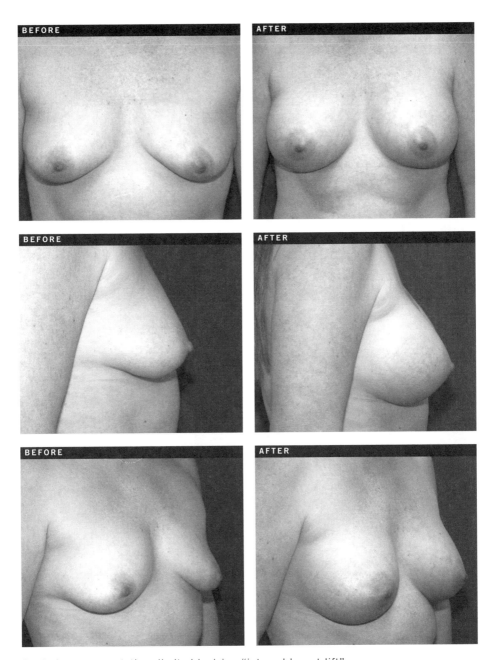

Dual-plane augmentation: limited incision "internal breast lift"

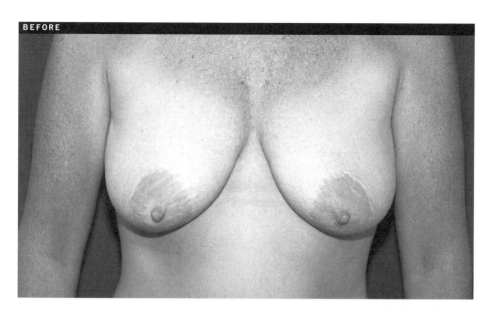

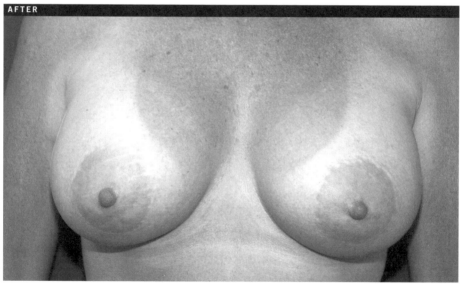

Dual-plane augmentation: limited incision "internal breast lift"

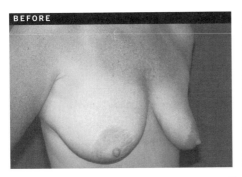
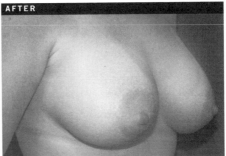

Dual-plane augmentation: limited incision "internal breast lift"

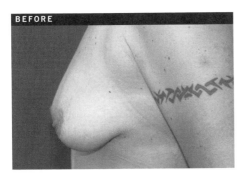
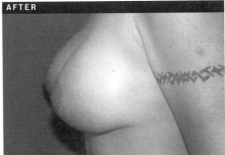

Dual-plane augmentation: limited incision "internal breast lift"

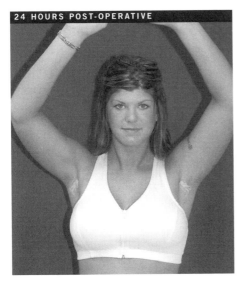

Patient doing arm exercises 24 hours after
rapid recovery breast augmentation

**After Surgery**

After your surgery, there are three very important things to do. The first is getting your arms over your head. You should begin to do this six to eight hours after surgery. Do a set of three arm raises every hour before going to bed. **The worst thing a marathoner can do after a race is to lie around doing nothing. Instead, stretching and walking help the muscles to recover more rapidly. The same principle holds true for the quick recovery method.** You may lift objects that weigh less than 30 pounds and drive a car if you're off prescription pain medication.

The second is actually a don't: Don't baby your breasts. You can't hurt or rupture your implants or rip open your stitches, a common but unnecessary fear, by going about your daily routine. Look at your breasts in a mirror. Touch them, and get to know them. They're not the same as what you've been used to all these years and they are going to feel weird for a while, so it's important to become familiar with them.

Finally, lie on your breasts—yes, that's right—for 15 minutes every day starting the evening of your surgery. Plan on doing this every day after surgery for one year. You will feel better and lessen the risk of developing scar tissue around the implant, which almost always occurs within one year.

**Road to Recovery**

You can and should go about your normal activities after your procedure. Your surgeon will give you guidelines regarding aerobic activities, dressings, and other issues at discharge time.

*"I was amazed at how quickly I recovered from my surgery,"* one patient said. *"I had the procedure done on Friday morning, and I was back at my desk at work on Monday morning. I was still a little sore, but I was able to get around just fine. Within two and a half weeks I was able to play softball."*

You should be able to return to work within a few days, depending on the activity level required for your job. Your breasts will be sensitive to direct stimulation for two to three weeks, so you should avoid physical contact during that time. Your scars will be firm and pink for at least six weeks. They may remain pink and the same size, or may even appear to widen, for several months. Your scars will never disappear completely but will **definitely fade and flatten over time.**

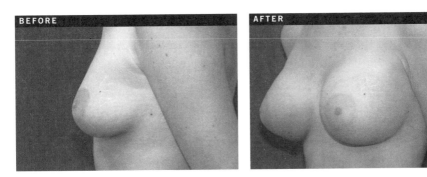

Breast augmentation to fill out the excess skin envelope

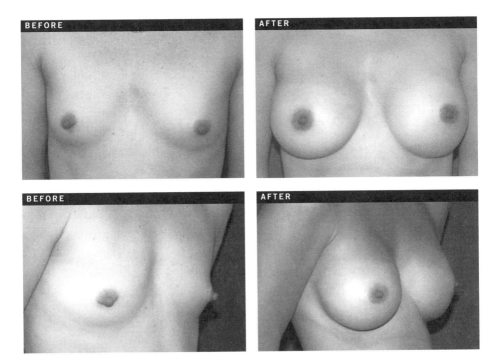

Breast augmentation in a patient who wanted her clothes to fit better

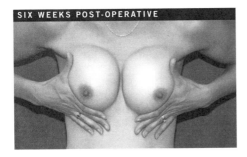

Same patient demonstrating implant softness

You may find that you feel a little depressed in the week or so following surgery. This is a normal reaction to the anesthesia and the changes your body has undergone. Just ride it out, and try not to worry about it too much. You will feel better soon.

When having mammography, notify the technician about the implants so additional views can be taken to examine the breast tissue more effectively. An implant will impair the accuracy of a mammogram to some extent. Choose a radiologist who is familiar with the special techniques that can enhance the results of the exam.

### Risks and Limitations

Implants can rupture. One patient asked why, wondering if the valve was the problem. Instead, a rupture is usually a small pinpoint leak that can develop on the implant's edge. **It's like an old sweater that has worn through the elbow while the buttons are holding just fine.** The implant's valve would be like the buttons—still working—while friction on the implant shell day in and day out can cause an area to spring a leak.

Many patients have the idea saline implants need to be replaced after a specific number of years. Automatic replacement must be necessary because the tabloids at the grocery store checkout line said so. Not really.

Your auto windshield only needs to be replaced if it is cracked, which is different from the routine maintenance to change your oil. Actually, there is no need to replace a saline implant unless it ruptures. I have patients whose implants have been fine for almost 20 years. I also have a small percentage of patients whose implants have ruptured and needed replacement.

Rarely, implants can become infected. It is extremely important to have surgery at an approved facility with flawless sterile technique. The most common complication of breast implants is excessive firmness, where the breast is harder than the patient or surgeon would like. This happens in about three to five percent of women following surgery in my experience. Nipple numbness occurs in about three percent of cases. I have patients sign an extremely long consent form, which lists virtually every known complication or adverse outcome.

In addition to those already mentioned, these could include:

- Capsular contracture—scar tissue around an implant that causes pain, firmness, and sometimes, a misshapen appearance.
- Calcification—calcium deposits that form in the tissue around an implant, causing hardening and pain.
- Wrinkling and folds—wrinkling or creasing of the implant surface that may result in irritation to surrounding tissue or deflation of the implant.

These all may sound scary, but complications are rare. Your surgeon can answer any questions you may have about the risks and can put them in perspective to ease your mind or help you decide not to proceed with surgery.

### When All Is Said and Done

As time goes by, your breasts will begin to feel more and more natural. Many women think they look better proportioned after breast augmentation. Friends and acquaintances may ask if you've lost weight (go ahead and tell them yes.)

*"A couple weeks after I had the surgery, I ran into some acquaintances who told me that I looked great and asked if I had lost weight or something,"* one of my patients said. *"I think what people are seeing is that I am now better proportioned, with my new bust making my hips look smaller. That was my goal in having the surgery. I didn't want to be really big, just proportioned to my hips."*

Your decision to have breast augmentation is a personal one, something you have done for yourself. If the surgery has met your expectations, that's all that matters.

*"I have spent the last 15 years being pregnant, raising kids, working, and taking care of everyone else but me,"* one woman said. *"Now I'm taking time to exercise and take care of myself, and the breast augmentation is part of my quest for self-improvement."*

## BREAST LIFT, OR MASTOPEXY

Mastopexy is a procedure to elevate the nipple-areolar complex and tighten the breast skin envelope. The procedure is used when the nipple height is approximately at or a bit below the breast crease, which often happens following childbirth or after breast-feeding. A very mild relaxation of the breast may be corrected with implants, by removing a crescent of skin from the upper half of the areola, or with the dual-plane breast augmentation procedure. When the nipple is well below the crease the breast laxity is more severe and will probably require additional incisions and skin removal. Breast implants inserted during a mastopexy can increase firmness and size.

Extremely large, heavy breasts—D cups or larger—tend to sag soon after a mastopexy, so women with larger breasts may not be good candidates for this surgery. The problem is that the skin envelope simply can't withstand the effects of gravity, although in some cases internal sutures, absorbable mesh, a muscle sling, or other techniques may be used to suspend the breast tissue. Pregnancy also may undo the positive effects of the surgery. Ideal candidates are women with moderate-sized breasts who are finished having children.

If there ever was a procedure that has to be tailored to the individual, it's mastopexy. Every patient's anatomy varies, so it is extremely important not only to be aware of all your options but also to discuss your procedure extensively with your surgeon.

Your surgeon will do a breast examination and take careful measurements of your nipples in relation to other parts of your breasts and your torso. Perhaps you'll only need a lift on one side. The size and shape you expect may not match what a surgeon has in mind, so bring in pictures to show your doctor what you envision. Your doctor should also give you a general idea of where your areola and nipple will be positioned.

Here are some things to consider when deciding whether to have a mastopexy:
- If your breasts differ markedly, do you want an enlargement or a reduction?
- How much scarring can you tolerate as a trade-off for a breast lift? Determine with your surgeon which lift procedure will give you the most improvement with the least scarring.
- Do you want a smaller areola? If so, how much smaller?
- Are you planning to have children or breast-feed children in the future? If so, your results may not last, and your surgery should be deferred until your family is complete.

Listen carefully to your surgeon's recommendations. Take notes if necessary. You're the one who has to live with the results.

When it comes to breast lifts, the most important element in patient satisfaction is realistic expectations. Remember that the results aren't permanent. Gravity, aging, and weight fluctuations can take their toll on your breasts again. Scarring will be considerable, even in "minimal incision" breast surgery. Be prepared for these outcomes before going ahead with a mastopexy.

**Mastopexy is very much a three-dimensional operation. If you combine it with breast augmentation, which is also highly three-dimensional, be prepared to experience some differences from one side to the other.** This may not happen, but the odds increase as you add two procedures together. Another possible complication when combining mastopexy with implants can occur if the muscle attachments are not properly released or the skin envelope isn't tightened. In this case the nipple can be forced downward, creating a "double-bubble" look as the breast hangs off the high-riding implant.

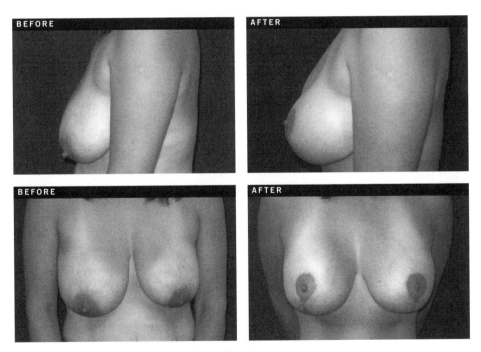

Breast lift with implants (side and front views)

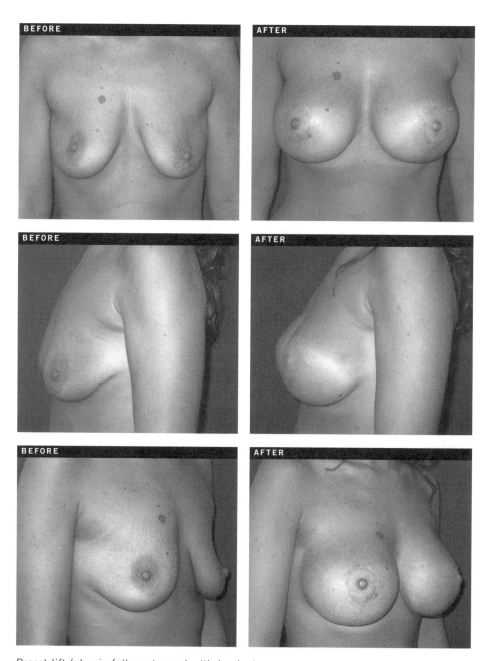

Breast lift (classic full mastopexy) with implants

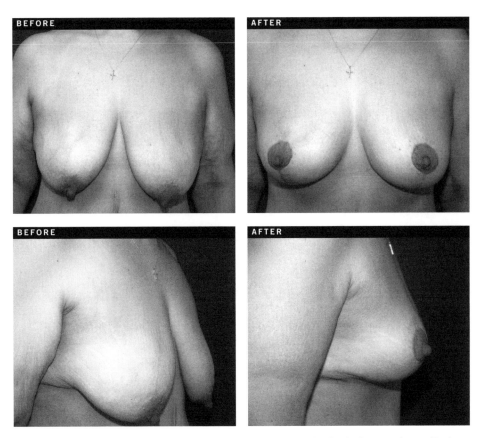

Classic mastopexy following massive weight loss in a post bariatric (stomach stapling) patient without implants

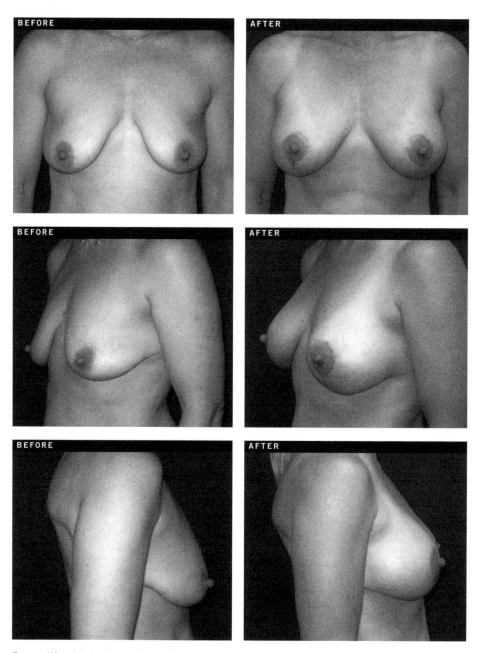

Breast lift with implants (multiple views)

## The Procedure

This is a same-day procedure usually done under general anesthesia but occasionally under intravenous sedation if limited incisions are to be used. The procedure takes about one and a half to three and a half hours. Depending on the nipple level and amount of excess skin, incisions can range from a small crescent above the areola to the classic incision pattern that looks like an anchor. I have created a procedure that uses a wavy incision around the areola, which can better camouflage the scar (published in *Plastic and Reconstructive Surgery*, 2002, p. 1778, "'Zigzag' Wavy-line Periareolar Incision"). Any of the mastopexy procedures may be done in combination with breast implants.

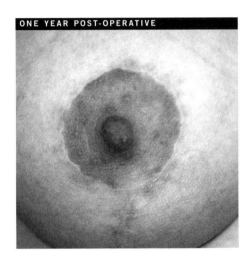

ONE YEAR POST-OPERATIVE

Mastopexy (breast lift): A "zigzag" wavy-line incision is made around the areola to create a more natural outer areolar border. Notice the gradually fading natural coloration one year after surgery.

*Crescent Mastopexy:* The most limited procedure involves removing a crescent or half-moon pattern of skin horizontally along the top of the areola. This leaves a curved scar along the top half of the areola. Crescent mastopexy can be used when the nipple needs to be raised about half an inch. It works well in combination with breast augmentation because the implant's volume also supports the nipple in an upward direction. Some surgeons prefer to place the implant on top of the muscle in a mastopexy procedure.

Note: This incision may "bottom out" a larger breast as the tightened upper breast pushes the still-relaxed lower breast down and out.

*Doughnut Mastopexy:* Doughnut or concentric mastopexy involves a circular incision around the nipple. A doughnut or ring of skin anywhere from one-half to two inches is removed. Upon closure the breast skin is tightened around the open doughnut as the nipple is elevated. This procedure is appropriate in a limited number of patients with smaller breasts and minimal sagging. It may flatten the breast slightly and can cause radiating folds of skin but avoids more extensive scars. Doughnut mastopexy may be extended with additional skin removal from below the breast. This helps support the breast upward.

*Classic Mastopexy:* This procedure has various forms. The most common follows the natural contour of the breast, with skin removed around the nipple, down the breast front, and horizontally along the crease. Internal tacking often is placed to support breast tissue higher on the rib cage. The nipple and areola are moved higher. Surrounding skin is pulled tight to shape and support the breast. This leaves an anchor-shaped incision.

A variation, known as minimal incision surgery, eliminates the incision across the breast crease. The smaller the breasts, the more minor the incisions.

## After Surgery

Your breasts will be bruised and swollen after surgery. Swelling will be minimal to moderate and last several weeks. Avoid salty foods to diminish excess swelling. Pain is moderate. Your surgeon will order pain pills and possibly an antibiotic. Stitches are buried and can be dissolvable, so no removal should be necessary. Some surgeons use permanent sutures which must be removed. Drains are rarely necessary. A drain is a small plastic tube connected to a light bulb shaped reservoir. The compressible reservoir creates gentle suction to remove excess fluid from the surgical area. The recovery room nurse will teach you how to care for the drain prior to your discharge from the surgery center.

Immediately after surgery, you may wear an elastic wrap or surgical support bra with gauze bandages. When you switch to a good support bra, wear it around the clock for three to four weeks. Avoid vigorous exercise or direct contact and avoid sleeping on your stomach for the same amount of time. Sexual activity that causes pain in the surgical area should be avoided.

Mild depression following surgery is normal, and is the result of the anesthesia. The best thing to do is ride it out—it will pass quickly.

Massive swelling on one side compared to the other, fever, redness, or unusual drainage are causes for alarm. Call your surgeon immediately.

### Road to Recovery

It is important to avoid lifting anything over your head for at least four weeks after a breast lift. The same holds true for engaging in strenuous exercise or sports. In rare cases, mastopexy could affect your ability to breast-feed. Subsequent pregnancies also may stretch your breasts to their pre-procedure sagging state, so many surgeons avoid performing a mastopexy until a woman has finished with child bearing.

### Risks and Limitations

There is a chance of numbness in the nipple or scattered areas of the breast skin. Bleeding can occur, even to the degree that a secondary drainage procedure can become necessary. As in any surgery, infection is possible. Incisions also could separate in high-tension areas. This usually requires cleansing and antibiotic ointment for several weeks as these areas heal.

Mastopexy leaves noticeable scars, which will be covered by your bra or bathing suit. If you smoke or don't follow recovery instructions completely, you're at risk for tissue death and scars that widen or become infected. The procedure also can leave unevenly positioned nipples and other breast asymmetries.

The major problem with breast lifts is that gravity keeps working, especially with women who have larger, heavier breasts. With newer techniques of suturing the internal breast tissue to the chest wall, longer-lasting results are available.

## BREAST RECONSTRUCTION

Awareness of the physical and psychological benefits of breast reconstruction surgery is growing, and more and more breast cancer patients are choosing to have this done. New surgical options are available, and advances in the field are helping surgeons create breasts that are softer, more natural looking, and more sensitive.

Patients whose breast cancer is detected at earlier stages are ideal candidates for breast reconstruction. New data also shows more women are choosing to have reconstruction at the time of a mastectomy, and "immediate reconstruction" now accounts for almost half of all procedures. Reconstruction does not increase the risk of breast cancer recurrence. If your oncologist recommends a mastectomy and you plan to have a reconstruction, ask for a referral to a plastic surgeon. In most cases breast reconstruction is covered by insurance.

## BREAST REDUCTION

Breast reduction patients are the happiest group of plastic surgery patients, studies show. These comments from patients help illustrate why:

*"I never really thought I was depressed about how large my breasts were,"* one woman wrote. *"As the date of my surgery came closer, I felt this great happiness. Now, four months later, I'm thrilled with the results and know this was one of the best decisions I have ever made."*

Another patient considered her breast reduction surgery results so natural:

*"I just forget I ever had the procedure. Imagine, after years of total body awareness, I could feel that comfort level."*

Women with heavy, pendulous breasts can suffer from a skeletal imbalance that contributes to back, neck, and shoulder pain. Some experience numbness in their hands and breathing problems due to nerve compression as their breasts pull down on their shoulders. Many women actually have grooves cut in their shoulders by their bra straps. They can develop a rash under their breasts, especially during warm weather. Psychologically, many patients have felt self-conscious about their breasts since they were young.

*"All my life I'd avoided any attention being drawn toward my breasts,"* one patient said.

Women having breast reductions usually are DD-cups or larger. The goal of the procedure is to relieve symptoms. The surgery is done for medical purposes, but appearance can be enhanced, too. Breast reduction or reduction mammoplasty involves removing excess fat, breast tissue, and skin. It's like a classic mastopexy except that volume is removed as well as excess skin. The areola is reduced, and a smaller, better-supported breast is constructed. The nipple is moved up. Occasionally, in women with very large breasts, the nipple-areolar complex may be completely removed and grafted onto the breast mound.

### Insurance Coverage

Insurance may cover breast reduction for some women. It depends on the patient's breast size, body type, and symptoms. Most insurance companies have a formula based on your height, your weight, and how much your surgeon estimates will be removed. Usually removal of about a pound from each breast is required for insurance coverage.

Health care providers are mercenary about denying coverage for breast reduction. They don't care if your clothes don't fit or you can't exercise. In my experience, they don't even care about your pain and discomfort, much less psychological embarrassment. It all boils down to your height and weight versus how much breast tissue will be removed. You can't necessarily pick your desired breast size or shape. To remove less than the insurance company's formula requires places the procedure in the realm of cosmetic surgery. That means you pay the bill.

Your surgeon should get a detailed medical history because some health-care providers demand a history of treatment for back pain to authorize coverage. I measure the breasts and often take photographs to be mailed with the insurance letter. If I don't comply with the rules, the insurance provider—who holds all the cards—may not authorize paying for the procedure.

### The Procedure

Usually, breast reductions are done as same-day surgery. They are done under general anesthesia and last two to three hours.

Techniques for breast reduction vary, but the most common procedure involves an anchor-shaped scar pattern. The incision surrounds the areola, proceeds down the breast's center, and ends slightly above the breast crease. Surrounding breast and subcutaneous tissue are removed along with excess skin, and the nipple and areola are raised to the level of the natural breast crease. The blood supply that originates from the chest wall to the areola is preserved. Skin is folded around the central breast tissue to form a new breast shape. Liposuction often is used to remove the excess roll on the side of the breast. This leaves a shorter scar than if the excess was surgically removed.

If the breasts are extremely large or if the nipples are very low, your surgeon may completely remove the nipple and graft it higher. If this is done, you will not have sensation in the nipple. Some surgeons try to eliminate the scar along the breast crease with a minimal incision approach. The problem with this approach is that it sometimes causes a puckering of the tissue at the base of the breast, which often requires revisional surgery.

Before deciding on a procedure, request photos of a surgeon's prior patients. This helps you understand what the scars will look like and roughly how big your breasts will be afterward. Photos really help settle a patient's mind and build realistic expectations. You may be shown videos and receive educational material. Your surgeon should describe the procedure in detail.

### After Surgery

I put my patients in a support bra following breast reduction. I sometimes use drains which are generally removed in a day or two. Buried sutures will dissolve on their own. Your breasts will be bruised and swollen for a week or two. Pain is moderate. Pain pills and possibly an antibiotic may be ordered.

You may feel a little depressed in the week or so following surgery. This is a normal reaction to the anesthesia and the changes your body has undergone, and shouldn't last long.

Patients should wear a bra day and night for the first month. They should avoid direct contact and sleeping on their stomachs. Swelling should be minimal to moderate and will last several weeks. Avoiding salty foods will reduce excess swelling. Patients should avoid vigorous activity for approximately one month after surgery.

### Risks and Limitations

Numbness in the nipple or breast skin can occur. Bleeding may occur that requires a secondary drainage procedure. Infection and separation of incisions in high-tension areas is possible. Blood can collect in the breast area, despite the use of drainage tubes. A small portion of skin or the nipple may die. Most patients are able to breast-feed after breast reduction surgery, but this cannot be guaranteed.

Definite postoperative scars are the trade-off for this surgery, although your clothing will hide them. Some women experience bad scarring or poor healing. This can be associated with smoking or even second-hand smoke, so don't smoke and take precautions if you think you might be exposed to second-hand smoke. Follow your surgeon's instructions to the letter.

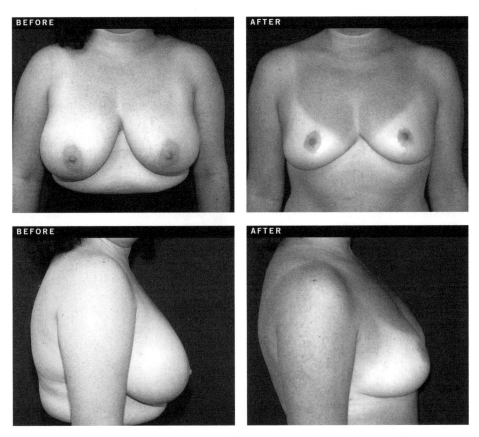

Breast reduction in a patient who returned for an abdominoplasty because "I can see my tummy now"

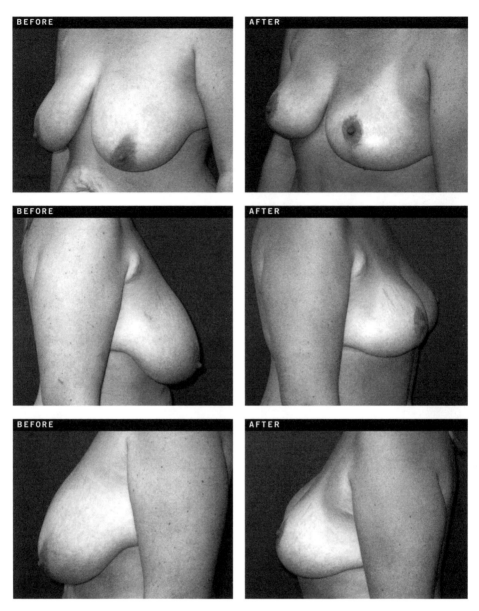

Breast reduction for back, neck and shoulder pain in a patient who had a tummy tuck and liposuction of the inner thighs during the same surgery

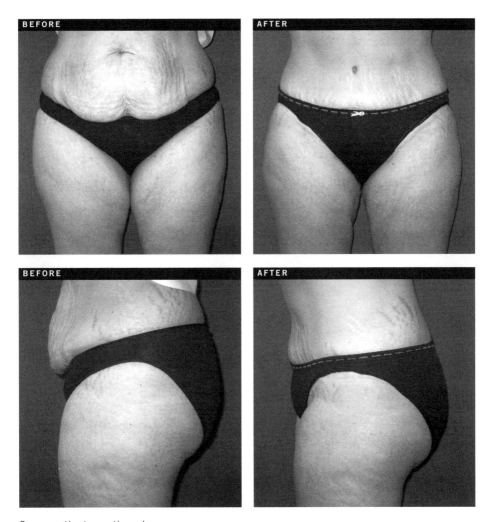

Same patient, continued

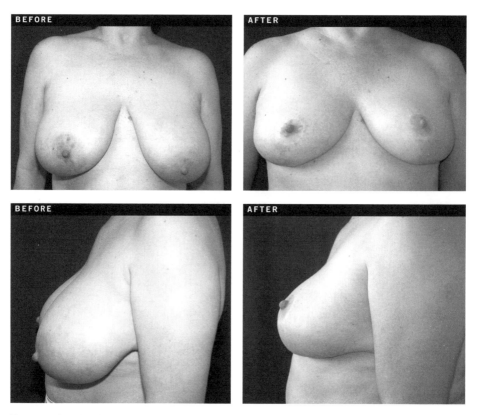

Breast reduction for large breasts which were affecting her posture and contributing toward back discomfort

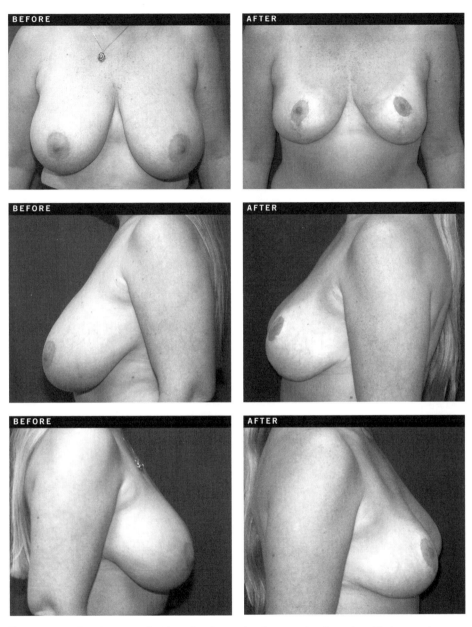

Three years after breast reduction showing natural appearing breasts with inconspicuous scars

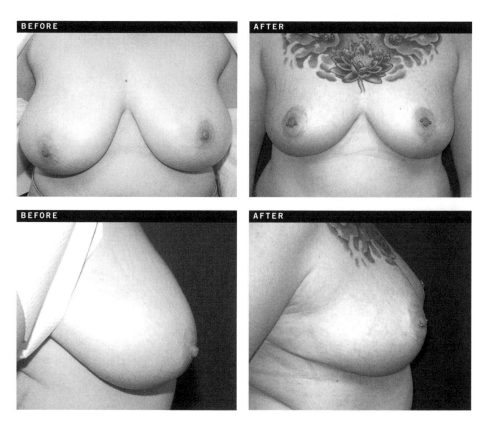

Three years postop breast reduction showing long lasting support - the tattoo did not come with the surgery

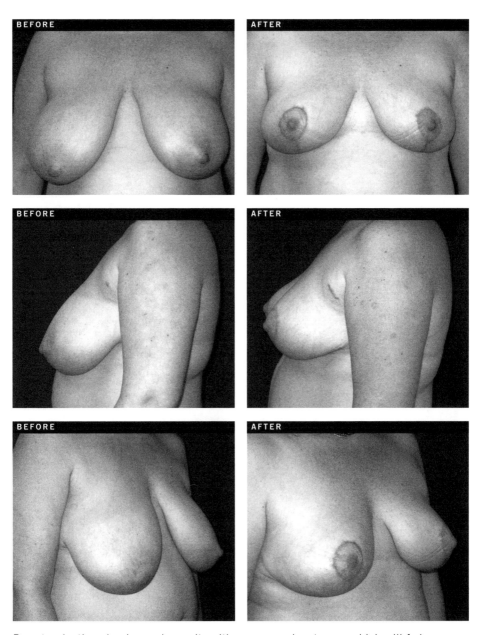

Breast reduction showing early results with more prominent scars which will fade over time

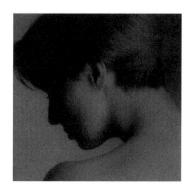

*chapter 7*

# RHINOPLASTY, FACELIFTS, AND OTHER FACIAL PROCEDURES

"Birthdays are only numbers…and mine's unlisted."

—Anonymous

## RHINOPLASTY, OR NOSE RESHAPING

*Rhino* means nose (like rhinoceros) and *plasty* means to shape, mold, or form. Rhinoplasty accounted for about two percent of all cosmetic surgery procedures in 2004, according to the American Society of Aesthetic Plastic Surgeons.

Many aesthetic plastic surgeons feel rhinoplasty is the most artistic and difficult cosmetic surgical procedure. I agree. Every change the surgeon makes has three-dimensional aspects that instantly alter other areas of the nose, like the ripple effect from a single stone cast into a quiet pond. As if that wasn't enough, the nose swells during the procedure, obscuring landmarks, and sometimes heals unpredictably. A limited number of experts specialize in rhinoplasty, so do your homework. With rhinoplasty, the touch-up rate is a solid 15 percent nationally.

In medicine, it is said that diagnosis is 50 percent of the cure. In rhinoplasty, accurate preoperative analysis is 50 percent of the outcome. Every nose is a completely different artistic adventure and the procedure must be individualized. Communication with the patient is essential. During patient consultations, I use photographs and a rhinoplasty diagram sheet to communicate clearly with the patient. I ask patients to pretend we have a surgical magic wand. I encourage them to bring in photographs of how they envision their result. One to three pictures is sufficient because any more can be confusing. I tell them, "I am an artist struggling to be a mind reader." The plan at the initial consultation is only a rough draft. I will refine this plan many times in my own mind before the actual day of surgery, like revising a term paper. There is an old saying in plastic surgery, "Measure seven times, but cut only once." All the steps of this plan are written out longhand and discussed in the preoperative area the day of surgery before we go into the operating room.

For some patients, I also have used computer imaging. An internal airway exam is a must to evaluate whether cartilage is present for grafting purposes from the septum or whether valve or airway problems exist. (If your surgeon fails to look inside your nose, you've visited an amateur.) As a patient looks in the mirror describing their concerns, I take precise and accurate notes. I see all my rhinoplasty patients at least twice before the procedure to be sure they have a clear understanding of goals and limitations.

*"My nose was kind of a non-issue,"* one woman patient said. *"It bothered me a little bit, but I always got over it and put surgery plans on the back burner. Then a special occasion would arise that we all like to capture on film. The camera couldn't conceal the crooked line in the middle of my face. I was finally ready to take the step. I was not going to get a new nose, just an improved and refined version of the one I was born with."*

In some patients who want smaller noses, grafting material may have to be added to refine their features. For instance, a patient may want the end of their nose to be smaller, saying, "I don't like the ball on the tip of my nose." However, removing the structural framework that creates the ball may cause the tip of their nose to drop down. Some patients initially say, "Hey, doc. You're not listening to me. I want my nose smaller, and you keep talking about adding more stuff to it." I know it sounds strange, but in some cases cartilage actually is added to refine the structure, support the skin, and fashion a better distributed nose, which then appears smaller.

**The Procedure**

Rhinoplasty is done on a same-day basis. I prefer general anesthesia because there tends to be bleeding in the back of the throat, and this may be a problem in a semiconscious patient. A breathing tube avoids this problem. I let patients make the final decision about anesthesia.

**After Surgery**

At the end of the procedure, I inject a long-acting numbing agent, so my patients leave the office pain free. Usually, a splint is placed on the nose and stays there for one week. Your nose will be noticeably swollen for several days. Don't blow your nose for about a week.

Some people feel a little depressed in the week or so following surgery. This is a normal reaction to the anesthesia and surgery, and should go away in a short time.

About half of my patients have bruising; the other half don't. It may take a year or more for all traces of swelling to go away, but you will definitely look better by the time the splint comes off a week after surgery.

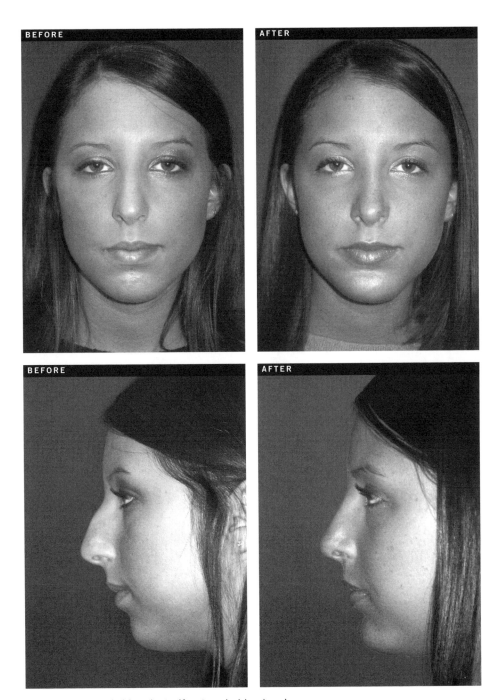

Chin implant and rhinoplasty (front and side views)

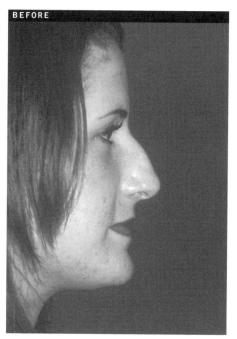
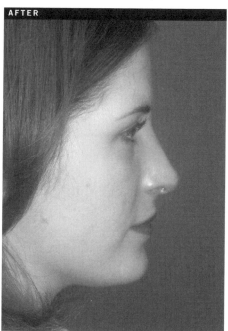

Rhinoplasty to reduce nasal hump

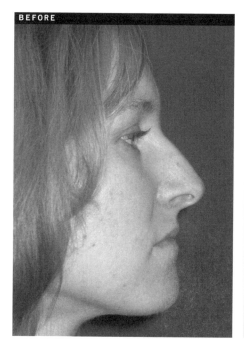
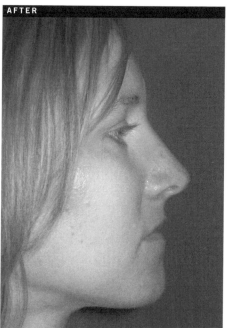

Rhinoplasty to refine bridge but preserve a strong profile

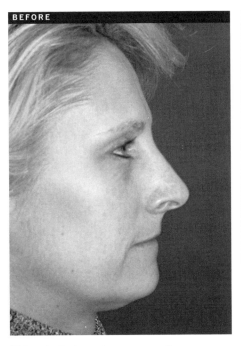

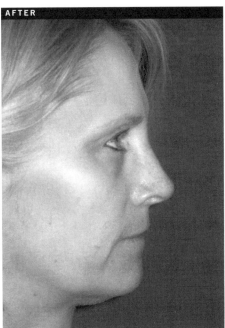

Rhinoplasty to make nose smaller

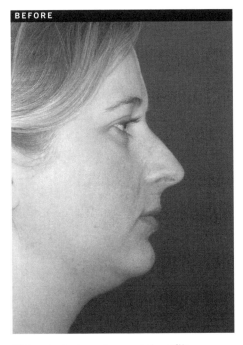

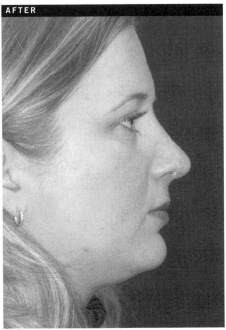

Rhinoplasty to reduce nasal profile

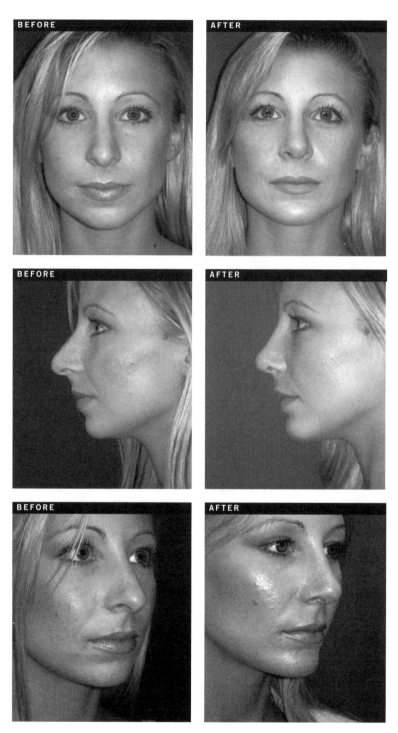

Chin implant (size: small) and open rhinoplasty for a patient desiring to refine and balance her features

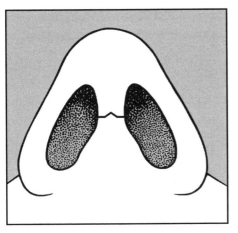

## OPEN RHINOPLASTY

Open rhinoplasty is often performed through an upside down "V" shaped incision underneath the nasal tip.

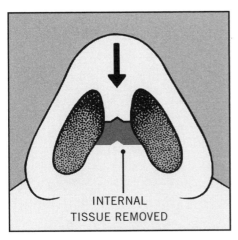

INTERNAL
TISSUE REMOVED

If the tip is long and the area around the incision is wide, the tip can be set back and narrowed.

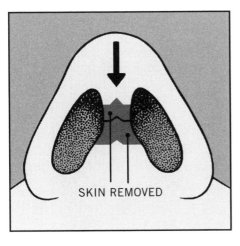

SKIN REMOVED

In extreme cases excess skin is removed below and even above the incision.

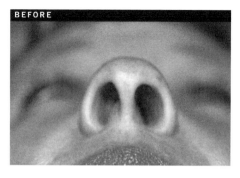

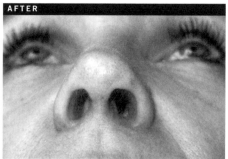

This patient underwent an open rhinoplasty to set back her tip and narrow her nostrils.

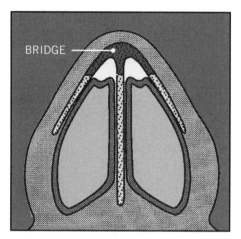

BRIDGE

## CLOSED RHINOPLASTY

Closed rhinoplasty is done through internal incisions. The bridge is identified through these internal incisions and trimmed to establish a pleasing profile.

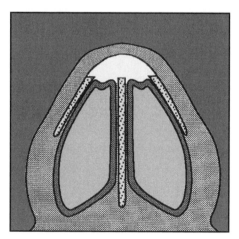

The bridge has been removed while protecting the inside lining of the nose. The internal incisions are then closed.

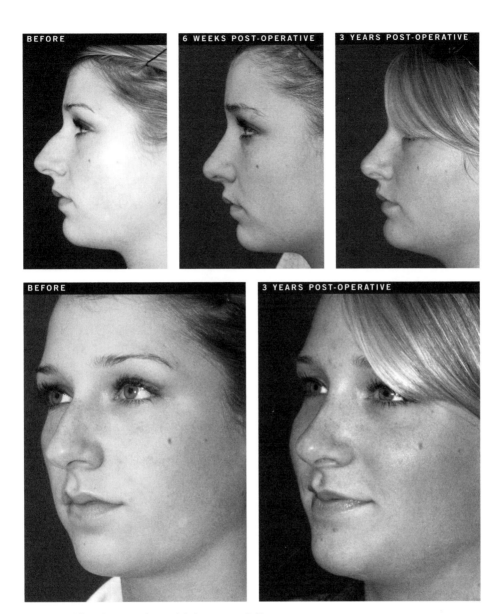

Teenage rhinoplasty patient with long-term follow-up

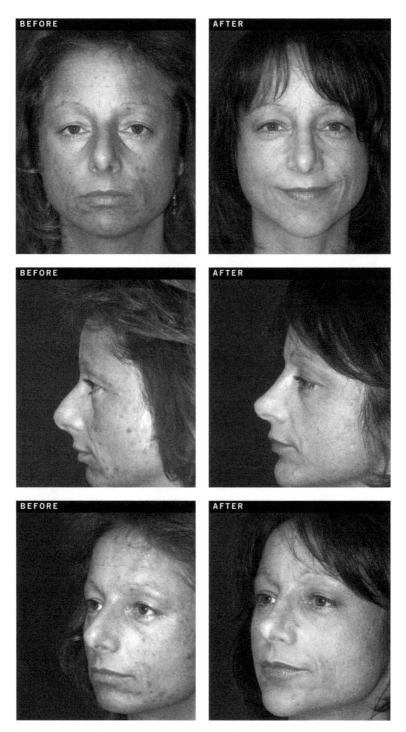

Chin implant with rhinoplasty showing multiple views one year postop

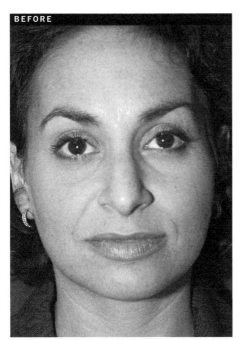

BEFORE

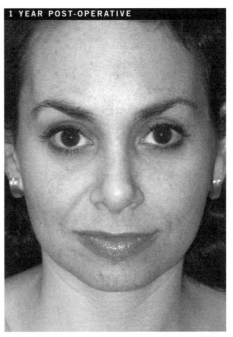

1 YEAR POST-OPERATIVE

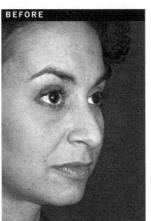

BEFORE

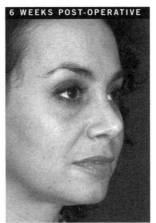

6 WEEKS POST-OPERATIVE

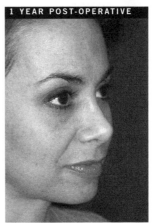

1 YEAR POST-OPERATIVE

Rhinoplasty (front and oblique views) to create a new tip

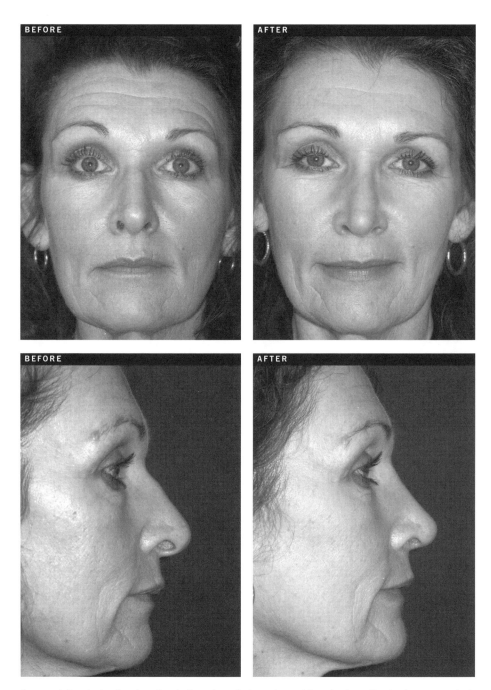

A complete study showing the full series of views in a rhinoplasty patient who requested hump removal and creation of an elegant profile

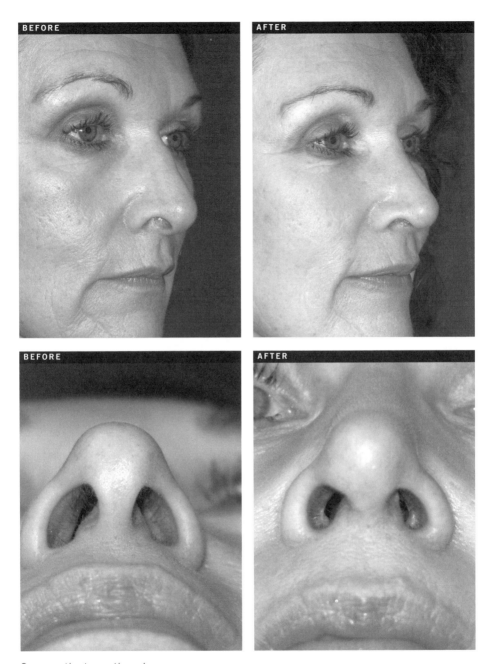

Same patient, continued

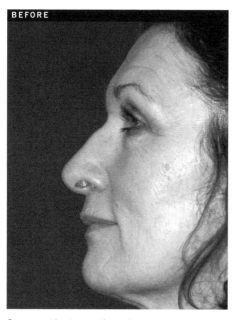 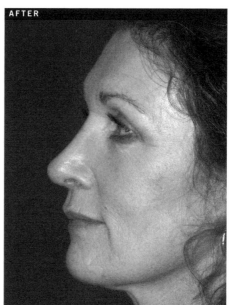

Same patient, continued

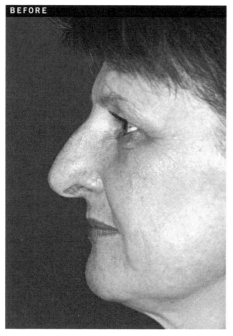 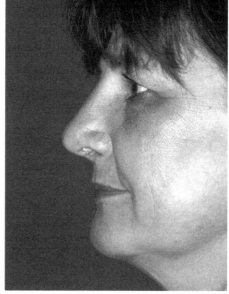

Rhinoplasty to rotate and set back nasal tip

## Risks and Limitations

Probably the biggest limitation with rhinoplasty is thick skin. Some noses have thick skin that will not shrink and conform to the underlying framework I fashion during the surgical procedure. A surgeon can do only so much with a large nose if the skin won't contract. Some patients with big noses and thick skin want a dainty small nose. I have to tell them, "I can't make a pup tent out of a circus tent."

Some risks include infection, postoperative nosebleeds, numbness, swelling, possible collapse of the nose, external scarring, skin loss, fullness, residual deformity, loss of the sense of smell, and holes inside the septal area of the nose. As always, the patient may not be satisfied, and revisional surgery may be needed. I can always find something to improve—a little too much of an angle here or a little dip there. I have never created, nor have I ever seen, a "perfect" nose.

## Aging Face
### vs.
### *Youthful Face*

---

long contours
vs.
*short contours*

narrow shape
vs.
*wide shape*

drawn
vs.
*full*

rectangular
vs.
*curved*

triangular
vs.
*heart-shaped*

long upper lip
vs.
*short upper lip*

thin, wrinkled lips
vs.
*smooth, full lips*

down-turned mouth
vs.
*up-turned mouth*

lower teeth show
vs.
*upper teeth show*

## FACELIFTS

Decades ago at a national convention, a New York plastic surgeon showed before and after photos of over a dozen facelift patients. Colleagues admired her surgical skill and impressive postoperative results. There was one catch. Toward the end of her talk, she explained that none of these patients had actually undergone a facelift procedure at all. They had been photographed standing upright in the "preoperative" photographs and lying on their backs in the "postoperative" photos. That's why grandma looked so good in her coffin.

As a person ages, the forehead increases in height, the nose drops, and the chin diminishes in size. People develop fullness along the jaw line, called a jowl, and neck skin migrates downward. When we lie down, gravity isn't pulling our faces downward. Instead, the jowl migrates back into the cheek area. Neck skin falls upward, which recreates a smoother neck angle and gives a more youthful look. Skin around the ear area also falls backwards.

At another meeting, one presenter showed a picture of himself standing on his head. The slide was projected upright, and he did indeed look much younger, particularly in the mid-face area. His deep cheek fold was shallower with a softer appearance. The cheek itself was located higher on the face and more toward the cheekbone. Lower eyelid bags were less apparent, and the upper lid skin and brows were elevated nicely. This physician had again demonstrated how surgery—or standing on your head—directly counteracts the aging effects of gravity.

In a matter of hours the clock is turned back and a patient's profile is transformed to a more youthful appearance.

*"I knew I wanted to look more refreshed, not different,"* one patient said. *"I felt young inside and felt I looked tired on the outside."*

The best candidate for a facelift has a face and neck that have begun to sag, good skin elasticity, and strong and well-defined bone structure.

Sometimes a patient fears that once she has one facelift, she will need another and another and another. I tell such a patient to imagine having an identical twin. If the patient has a facelift she will always look seven to ten years younger, on average, than her twin. The result of a facelift is permanent, but you will still continue to age normally. However, you will look better at any given age than if you had not undergone the procedure.

### Avoiding the Extreme Facelift

We've all seen Hollywood stars with overly taut facial skin from two or three facelifts. The best way to avoid the extreme-facelift look is to see a skilled practitioner who has done a lot of facelifts. Look at patient photos, and check out the results. Do any of the faces look overdrawn and tight? If so, seek your surgery elsewhere.

Discuss your concerns about the tight look with your surgeon. An overdone look may actually be secondary to over-elevated eyebrows, which results in a surprised or shocked look. It's very rare to have an overly tight look from a first-time facelift. Overly tight skin comes about when a facelift is redone.

Plastic surgeons who commonly do facelifts are aware of this problem and take measures to prevent it by not removing or resecting too much skin. Instead, they concentrate on supporting the deeper facial structures. Supporting this deep structure generally gives longer-lasting results, and may postpone some of the signs of aging for up to fifteen years.

One of the key elements to preventing an over-corrected facelift is to pull different areas of the face in different directions. Within each layer of the facelift procedure, different vectors (directions of force) of pull are established to allow a more natural look. The middle part of the face ages almost straight down, whereas the jaw line needs to be elevated at more of an angle to establish a youthful look. The overlying cheek skin is moved to the side. Overall, the facial appearance should be softer than it was before surgery.

One analogy is that of a bedspread. When making a bed, the appearance is improved simply by pulling up on the bedspread. However, to achieve the best result, you must rearrange all of the covering layers—the sheet, the blanket, and the bedspread—and straighten them in the proper direction for each one.

### The Procedure

Facelifts used to be performed by elevating the skin over the facial area, pulling it upward, removing the excess, and closing the incisions, but current practice now involves extensive work on the deeper facial structures. Some of the procedures used in facelifts are extremely difficult and not meant for every practitioner. Discuss the type of approach your surgeon would use and be sure to find a surgeon with plenty of training and experience in the procedure.

Many facelifts are performed under local anesthesia combined with a sedative. This means you will be awake but relaxed and without pain. An alternative is to have the surgery done under general anesthesia. Either one is perfectly acceptable. Talk it over with your surgeon to find the best option for you.

A facelift usually takes several hours to perform. Incisions begin above the hairline at the temples, extend down the natural line in front of the ear, and continue behind the earlobe to the lower scalp. Skin is separated from fat and muscle below, and those tissues are trimmed, suctioned, incised, and tightened as needed. Skin then is pulled back over the face, and the excess is removed.

## Signs of a Bad Facelift

- Tension lines

- Skin pleats

- Distorted mouth

- Startled brow

- Hairless scalp incisions

- Sideburns displaced upward

- Attached earlobes or "pixie ears"

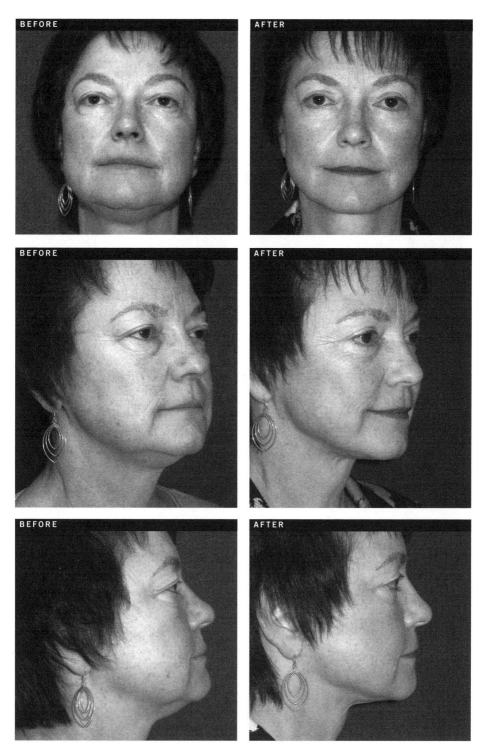

Facelift patient 18 months postop

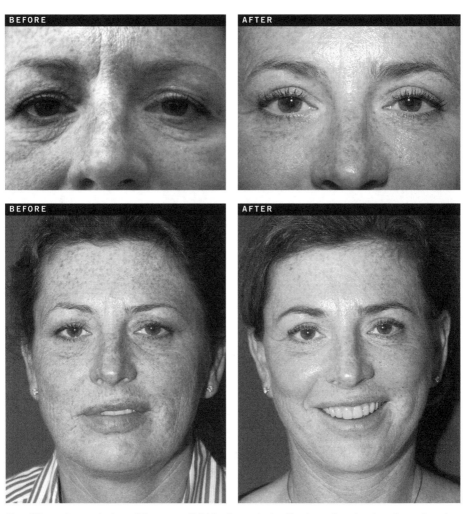

Facelift, endoscopic browlift, upper lid blepharoplasty, lipotransfer cheeks, dermabrasion upper lip, and lower lid skin excision – three months postop

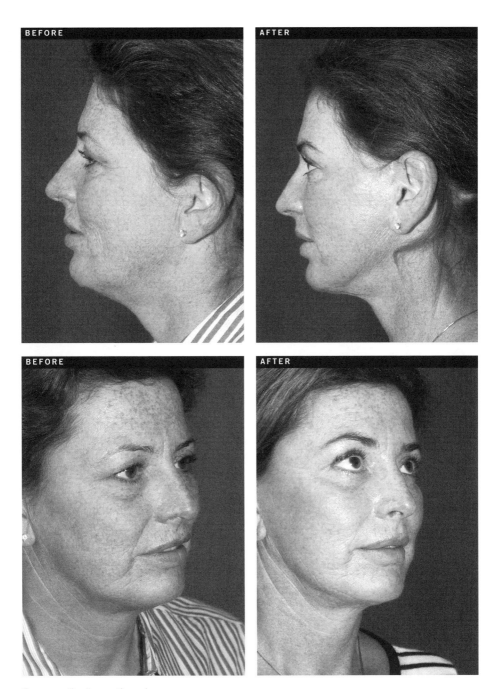

Same patient, continued

The incisions of a facelift may be brought into the hairline or may be behind the ear or even on the front side of the ear, depending on the surgeon's and patient's preference. An incision can be made along the lower edge of the sideburn area to keep this hair from shifting upward as skin is pulled up from the neck. Discuss precisely where the surgical incisions will be made and make certain your surgeon's preference is clear, along with alternatives, so you can come to an agreement on the incisions and the type of facelift that best suits your particular anatomy. Most facelift surgeons customize their procedure to some degree depending on the individual patient.

## NECK LIPOSUCTION WITHOUT FACELIFT

Patients with neck fullness may not be candidates for a face lift because of medical conditions, high blood pressure, smoking, blood thinning medications, or patients may disqualify themselves because of cost, unavailable recovery time, or emotional resistance to "such a big procedure." I have published a six-year study involving 132 patients who had neck liposuction without a facelift (published in *Plastic and Reconstructive Surgery,* 2003, p. 1393, "Submental Suction-Assisted Lipectomy without Platysmaplasty: Pushing the (Skin) Envelope to Avoid a Facelift for Unsuitable Candidates"). Neck liposuction without a facelift was observed to be a reasonable alternative for some patients who were unable or unwilling to undergo a facelift.

Localized fullness in the middle of the neck was observed to be the best predictor of a good outcome. A crepe paper appearance of the skin preoperatively was the best predictor of failure. I still advise healthy older patients intent on reliable definitive changes to undergo a facelift. More about liposuction in general is discussed later in this book.

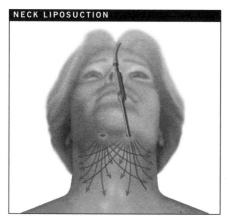

NECK LIPOSUCTION

Illustration of cross-tunneling

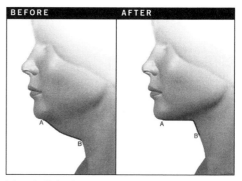

BEFORE    AFTER

Line A–B is the same distance in each photo

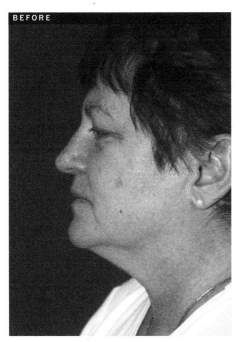
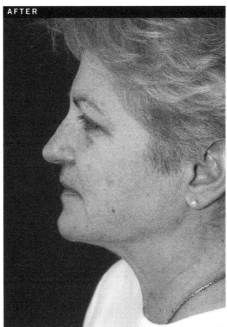

Neck liposuction without facelift

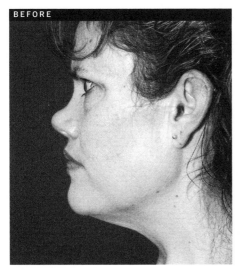
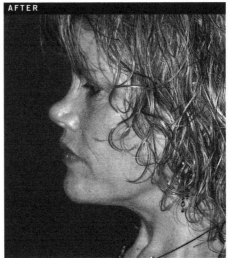

Liposuction neck without facelift, and lower lid blepharoplasty

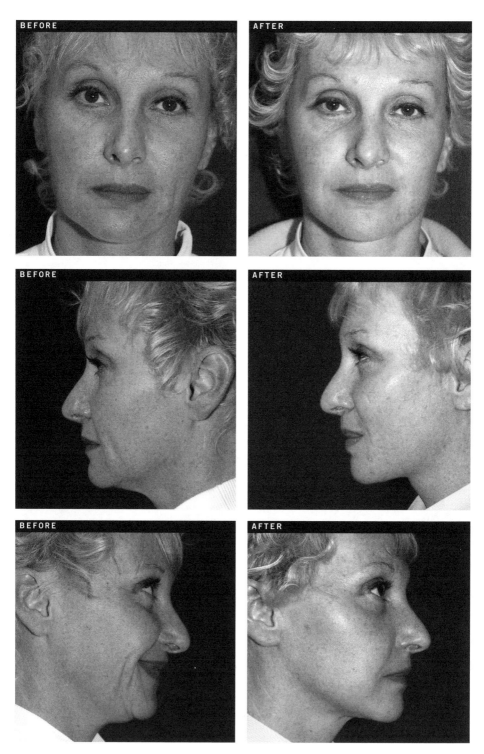

Minimal incision facelift ("mini-lift") – note how smiling accentuates excess neck skin

## MINIMAL INCISION FACELIFT

The minimal incision facelift, also known as the *short-scar facelift* or *mini-lift*, has been gaining popularity in recent years. It combines lipoplasty with less invasive surgical procedures than those used in a traditional facelift. The smaller incision used in this procedure produces about 50 percent less scarring than traditional facelifts. This is great for the patient, but performing in minimal quarters requires maximal skill from your surgeon. Be sure to choose someone with plenty of experience with this demanding procedure. The best candidates for the minimal incision facelift are usually younger patients with good skin elasticity.

### After Surgery

After the facelift is completed, the incision is sutured and a dressing is applied. A small, thin tube may be inserted to drain excess blood. I usually use a drain on my patients and wrap them up like a mummy overnight. Discomfort after a facelift is usually minimal and can be managed with minor pain medication. Some facial numbness is normal and will disappear in a few weeks to a few months. To keep swelling down, it's important to keep your head elevated when you're reclining for a week or two following surgery.

I always see my facelift patients the day after surgery, even if it's Saturday. If you have a drainage tube, it will be removed then, along with any bandages. Your face will look bruised, puffy, and pale, but will improve daily as recovery progresses. Stitches will be removed after about five days. Incisions in your scalp will take longer to heal and those stitches or clips may be left in a few days longer. Bruising is present for anywhere from 10 to 21 days, and often the patient looks fine with makeup as soon as seven days postoperatively.

### Road to Recovery

Take it easy for about a week after a facelift. Avoid strenuous exercise, sex, and heavy housework for at least two weeks. Also steer clear of alcohol, steam baths, and saunas. Limit sun exposure—which you should be doing anyway—for several months. Get plenty of rest.

In the first weeks after surgery, your face may look and feel strange. There will be bruising and swelling. Facial movements may feel stiff. Some patients get the blues after any procedure, but this is especially common after a facelift. This is the result of a biochemical letdown, partially from the anesthesia and perhaps also as a result of the change in your appearance. Just ride it out, like a surfer gliding on a small wave. Your negative feelings will go away in a few days. You can buy special makeup to cover the bruising, and by the third week you should look and feel much better.

### Risks and Limitations

Skin loss from smoking or other nicotine use is a serious risk for facelift patients. I can't stress enough how important it is to quit smoking before the procedure. I won't do a facelift on a smoker who won't—or can't—quit. If patients tell me they're going to quit, I try to believe them, but unfortunately people are not always honest with me, or maybe with themselves. Using nicotine products or even coming in contact with second-hand smoke can cause serious complications that can affect your appearance forever. Wait to have this procedure until you truly have quit.

Complications from a facelift can include infection, hematomas (a collection of blood under the skin), elevation of the hairline, baldness, skin loss or tissue death, delayed healing, skin numbness, ear numbness, facial weakness, and bad scarring. Rarely, prolonged or permanent pain or uncomfortable sensations have been reported in facelift patients. As with all procedures, a patient may not be satisfied with the results and may need revisional surgery.

High blood pressure can cause bleeding during and after surgery, sometimes necessitating an unexpected return trip to the operating room. I treat elevated blood pressure aggressively, and we will work with your family physician to lower even borderline blood pressure for two weeks before and after surgery to keep it below 140 over 90. As with all surgeries, complications can be caused by blood thinning medicines and herbs, which should be avoided for two weeks before and after surgery.

### When All Is Said and Done

A facelift turns back the clock, but it doesn't stop it. You may wish to have the procedure repeated five or ten years down the line. However, the effects of even one facelift are long lasting, and you should be happier with your appearance than if you hadn't had a facelift at all.

## FOREHEAD LIFT

Drooping eyebrows may lead a patient to seek a forehead lift, also called a browlift. This procedure restores the eyelid area to a more youthful oval shape. A forehead lift may require surgery to remove and tighten excess tissue, or it may simply involve releasing muscles that cause frown lines—the lines parents often get when giving "The Look" to their children.

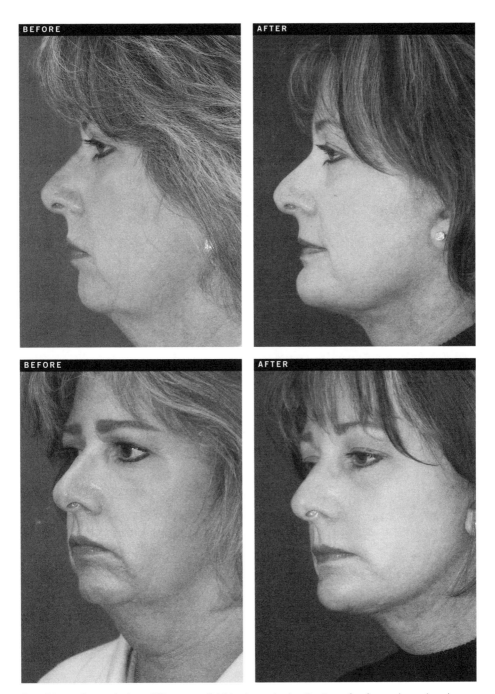

Facelift, endoscopic browlift, upper lid blepharoplasty, lipotransfer face, dermabrasion upper lip, chin implant

For a better understanding of how this procedure might change your appearance, look into a mirror and place the palms of your hands at the outer edge of your eyes, above your eyebrows. Gently draw the skin up to raise the brow and forehead area. This is approximately what a forehead lift would do for you. If you think this makes you look shocked or surprised, you probably shouldn't have a forehead lift.

I take great care to mark my patient's skin preoperatively while they look in a mirror and verify their preferred brow placement. This allows me to accurately replicate the direction of pull and determine how much elevation is necessary.

## The Procedure

Most forehead lifts are done through three or four small scalp incisions, each less than an inch long. An endoscope, a tiny, pencil-like camera, is inserted through one of the incisions. While looking through the endoscope, the doctor inserts an instrument through a second incision and lifts the skin and muscle. At the same time, the surgeon removes or alters underlying tissues. Eyebrows also may be lifted and secured into a higher position by sutures beneath the skin's surface. Occasionally, an incision is made across the top of the head from ear to ear, all hidden in the hair. This may be a more reliable approach depending on how thick and heavy the brow is.

## After Surgery

You may experience some numbness, incision discomfort, and mild swelling after your surgery. Pain at the incision site is usually minimal, and mild pain medication can manage it. Stitches or staples will be removed within one week. Temporary fixation screws will be removed in two weeks, if they were used.

## Road to Recovery

It's a good idea to take it easy the week after your surgery. You should be able to shower and shampoo your hair within two days. Most patients are back at work in a week. Vigorous physical activity should be limited for a couple of weeks. Limit exposure to heat and sun, which may promote swelling.

Scars from your forehead lift should fade quickly, but they are permanent. Although you may feel a little down at first, your mood will improve as your body chemistry gets back in sync and you look and feel better.

### Risks

Risks involved with forehead lifts are minimal, but can include temporary injury to the nerves that control eyebrow movement, infection and bleeding, delayed healing, and numbness. As with a facelift, high blood pressure can cause complications. Any elevation in blood pressure is treated with a long-lasting antihypertensive pill preoperatively.

### When All Is Said and Done

As with a facelift, a forehead lift is a procedure you may have to repeat in the distant future. However, you should be pleasantly surprised at how such a simple procedure can take years off your face.

## MID-FACE LIFT

A mid-face lift elevates the cheeks and tissue from the lower eyelid down to the corners of the mouth. A traditional facelift, which deals with the neck and jaw line, doesn't lift tissue as well in this area.

### The Procedure

Most surgeons make an incision below the lash line of the lower eyelid, and then go below the bone lining, called the periosteum. This incision travels down over the cheekbone and eventually breaks through the periosteum in the soft tissue under the cheek fold. Pulling on this segment will raise the corner of the mouth. It may be necessary to shore up the eye as well. A second, and my preferred, approach is to avoid the lower lid incision and use an endoscope inserted through the scalp to guide an incision hidden behind the hairline along the side of the temple area and down into the cheek. A second incision is hidden inside the mouth. Sutures are placed in the cheek tissue and passed up to the scalp area to suspend the midface from above the temple area. The sutures dissolve after about six months.

### Risks and Recovery

Risks and recovery for a mid-face lift are similar to those of a regular facelift. A mid-facelift can also be performed during a standard facelift procedure.

## DERMABRASION

Dermabrasion uses a high-speed rotating diamond brush on the facial skin, causing a controlled abrasion injury that subsequently heals. This works for smoothing the skin to lessen acne scarring, fine lines, or irregularities. Dermabrasion is an in-office procedure often done by dermatologists, and I use dermabrasion for the fine lines around the mouth when I am doing a combined facial procedure.

### Risks

The risks include prolonged redness or itching, possible scarring, and color changes.

## BLEPHAROPLASTY, OR COSMETIC EYELID SURGERY

Do you always look tired? Do you have folded or wrinkled upper eyelid skin? Drooping eyebrows? Pouches under your eyes? Eyes have been called the windows of the soul. They often are what people first notice about us. If someone wants advice about their aging face and asks whether to get a facelift or an eyelid tuck, I always say, "eyes first." They bespeak our age more readily than any part of the face.

Blepharoplasty is a surgical procedure to remove excess upper or lower eyelid skin and fat. In addition to the affect on appearance, drooping eyebrows and upper lids may be associated with vision impairment.

If skin resting on the upper eyelashes restricts a person's vision, an upper lid blepharoplasty may be covered by insurance. It will be necessary for your doctor to send a letter requesting prior authorization for this procedure with a photograph demonstrating the extent of the deformity and results of a visual field exam, which will be done by an eye doctor.

Eyelid surgery will not remove fine smile lines or widespread crepe paper skin, both of which can be treated by peels, laser surgery, or Botox injections. Lower eyelid surgery has little effect on dark circles, which can also be treated with bleaching creams, peels, or lasers. Some people of Asian descent want eyelid surgery to make them look more European. This surgery can establish an upper lid fold, but beyond adding the crease will not change other ethnic features.

Expectations are everything. Don't bring in photos of models who are smiling, yet have no facial wrinkles. Often photos of models are touched up—an illusion. Photos such as these shouldn't be a standard for a post-operative result.

An eyelid tuck might make you feel younger and more confident, but you have to have realistic expectations. Most people who undergo blepharoplasty

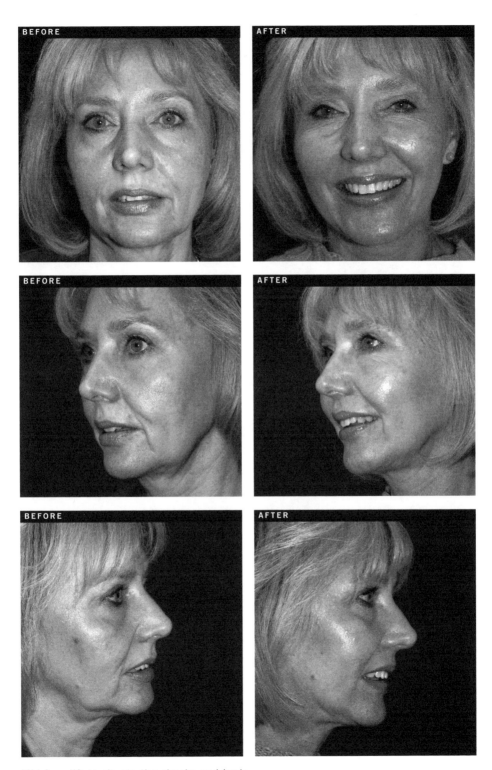

Mid-face lift to elevate the cheeks and jowls

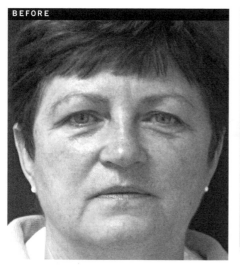
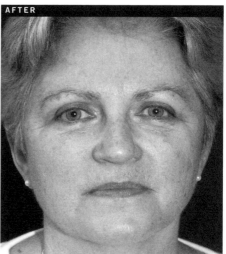

Four lid blepharoplasty

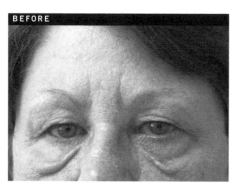
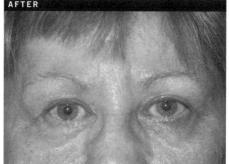

Eyelid tuck and excision of cheek bags

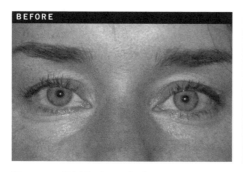
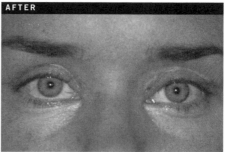

Upper eyelid blepharoplasty

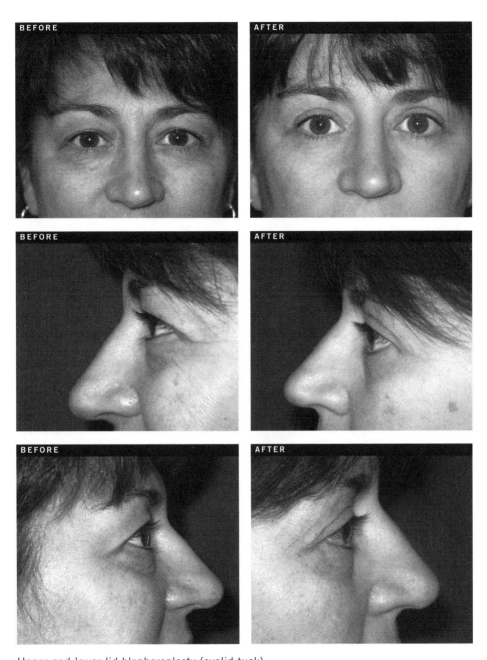

Upper and lower lid blepharoplasty (eyelid tuck)

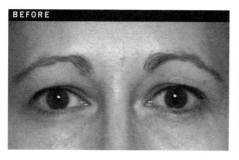
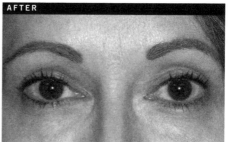

Upper lid blepharoplasty to remove familial excess skin

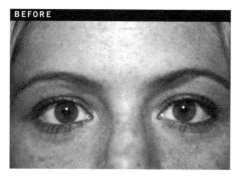
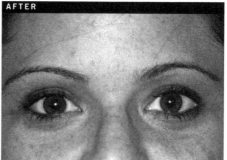

Upper lid blepharoplasty to remove excess skin in this young adult

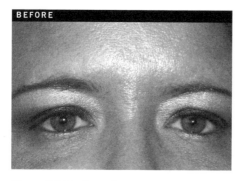
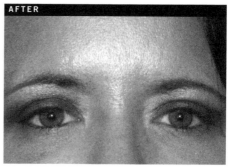

Upper lid blepharoplasty to remove excess skin resting on her eyelashes

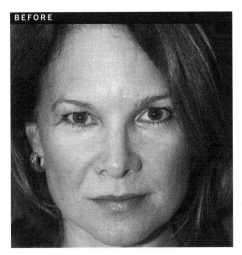

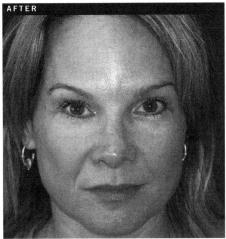

Brow lift and upper lid blepharoplasty one year postop

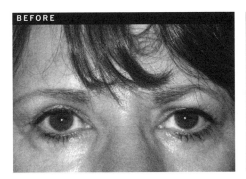

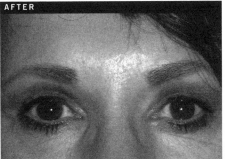

Preop and postop open brow lift

are in late middle age when they notice some bagginess under the lower eyelids and at the inner corners of the upper lids. This is caused by protrusion of the fat pads under the eyelid skin. This tendency can run in families and may become noticeable at an early age. Sometimes it's even evident in high school graduation pictures. For most people, however, fullness usually appears during middle age and beyond.

Blepharoplasty may be done with other cosmetic procedures. Botox injections, laser surgery, or dermabrasion for the fine lines around the mouth are the most common adjunct procedures done with eyelid tucks. Drooping brows may need to be corrected with a browlift. A facelift, browlift, and blepharoplasty are a frequent "blue-plate-special" for across-the-board facial rejuvenation. Botox injections put icing on the cake.

### Preparing for Surgery

You must provide an accurate health history for your surgeon to judge your suitability for a blepharoplasty. At your consultation you should be able to look in a mirror and explain your concerns exactly to your surgeon. Your goals and expectations should be clearly and openly discussed.

A surgical plan needs to be formulated that answers the following questions:
- Should all four lids or only the uppers or lowers be done?
- Will my lower eyelid incision be done internally or externally?
- Is the lower lid tone weak, necessitating a suspension procedure?
- Do I have a low tear level that may preclude doing all four lids at once?
- Do I want to elevate the outside attachment of my eyelids to give them a slight tilt upwards?
- Will skin as well as fat be removed?
- Are any additional procedures appropriate, such as a browlift, Botox, or even a mid-face lift?

During your visit, a tear production test and a general vision exam may be performed. Your plastic surgeon will want to know about your last eye examination, especially any physical findings, to determine if you are a good surgical candidate. You may be asked about glaucoma, contact lenses, high blood pressure, and thyroid disease.

The surgeon will examine the tone of your lower lids, possibly pinching and pulling down the skin to judge its ability to "snap back." Close-up preoperative photos will be taken, and computer imaging may be offered to you. I hold back the extra upper eyelid skin with a bent paper clip and gently push in the lower lid fat pads with a cotton swab to give an accurate impression of postoperative appearance.

Be sure to ask any questions you might have and make your expectations clear, because blepharoplasty is highly individualized surgery. You might also discuss the possibility of a browlift rather than an eyelid lift with your surgeon. Sometimes upper eyebrow laxity rather than excess upper lid skin may be the real culprit in drooping eyelids. Occasionally, a browlift along with an eyelid tuck may be your best solution.

**The Procedure**

Surgery is done on a same-day basis, taking anywhere from thirty minutes to two hours. Normally, you will be sedated. Numbing drops are placed in each eye, then local anesthesia is used to numb the area around the eyes. I prefer to keep patients heavily sedated during injections. From then on, you won't feel any pain but may feel some tugging. Once the injections are given, you can be less sedated if you prefer. General anesthesia is always an option.

On the morning of surgery, I have my patients again verify the surgical plan and confirm the placement of all incisions while looking in a mirror. This gives us a chance to discuss any last-minute questions or concerns. Your upper eyelid skin will be pinched to determine how much can be removed safely. Fat pads on your lower lids will be marked as you are asked to gaze in different directions. Slight pressure may be applied to your eye to make any fatty excess more obvious for the surgical outline.

The upper eyelid incision will be made slightly below the natural crease or very near to it. It will be carried out to the side within a smile line to better camouflage the scar. A crescent of excess eyelid skin will be removed. I generally don't excise any muscle. When appropriate, both fat pads are trimmed back very conservatively to prevent a sunken eye appearance.

The lower lid incision may be made on the inside of the eyelid. Some surgeons believe this preserves lower lid tone. An external incision can interrupt the lower lid's support system, causing relaxation—a sort of hound-dog look—in years to come. An internal incision, called transconjunctival, avoids an external scar. However, if you have excess lower-lid skin a pinch of external skin may have to be removed, which can be done without cutting into the muscle. The external scars are very inconspicuous. Eyelid skin is the thinnest on the body, making it the most forgiving when it comes to scarring.

Through either the internal or external approach, the three fat pads in each lower lid will be identified and trimmed as appropriate. A suspension procedure to support your lower lid or enhance the attachment of the outside corner of your eye may be done.

External eyelid incisions may be closed with stitches under the skin, called subcuticular sutures. Adhesive skin closure tape may be applied. Some surgeons prefer a running outside suture or dissolving sutures. Internal incisions may be closed with absorbable sutures or simply left open to allow for drainage. Another procedure such as a peel may be done immediately following your blepharoplasty for fine skin lines.

### After Surgery

Following surgery, you should experience only mild discomfort. Pain medication will be prescribed. If you develop loss of vision or pain in the eyeball itself, as opposed to the incision, call your doctor immediately. You will receive postoperative instructions that you should follow carefully. You will want to elevate your head when reclining and use ice packs. You could do paperwork or watch television the following day but should avoid vigorous activity for two to three weeks.

Ask your doctor when you can wear contact lenses. I have soft contact wearers wait about one week and hard contact wearers about two weeks, depending on the procedure. Using a special plunger to insert and remove your lenses will allow you to use them much sooner. Skin tapes and sutures are removed anywhere from three to five days after surgery. Bruising may be apparent for 10 to 21 days but can be concealed easily with makeup after a week has passed. You may develop transient sun sensitivity or excess tearing, which dark glasses will mollify.

You may feel a little depressed after your surgery. This is a normal biochemical reaction to the surgery and the anesthesia, and should go away in a few days.

### Risks and Complications

You should be in good health to have this surgery. A history of dry eyes, dry mouth, or joint aches from diagnosed arthritis may signal a connective tissue disease that would increase your risk of dry eye problems. Thyroid disease may cause the eyeball to protrude, forcing the lower lids downward and sometimes causing spasms in the upper lids. Low thyroid function could inhibit tear production.

Uncontrolled high blood pressure may cause bleeding during or after the operation. Any elevation in blood pressure is treated with a long-lasting antihypertensive pill preoperatively, and we will work with your primary care physician to keep your blood pressure under 140 over 90 for two weeks before and after surgery. If you have ongoing eye problems such as glaucoma, a detached retina, or recent eye surgery, including Lasik surgery, your ophthalmologist would have to clear you for blepharoplasty. People with uncontrolled diabetes or cardiovascular disease may have problems with such an operation.

Risks with this procedure in the upper eyelids include a "dog ear," which is an area of fullness at the end of the incision. Another problem I've seen in a couple of my patients over the years is prolonged swelling on one side as opposed to the other. The main risk with lower lid procedures is muscle laxity that causes the lid to pull down. It's best to diagnose this prior to the surgery and take steps to alleviate it during the cosmetic procedure. You might experience eye irritation or even cloudy vision from your prescribed eye ointment for a few days. Whiteheads may occur along your upper lid incision, but your surgeon or a nurse can remove them easily.

If you are undergoing an upper lid tuck, you may not be able to completely close your eyes for a week or two. Spouses usually notice this, joking that they're being watched even while the patient is asleep. However, if the lid is open an eighth of an inch or so, just the right amount of skin has been removed to give a clean upper lid crease. As swelling decreases, the lid assumes its normal position. Rarely, a patient's upper lids may never completely close, causing dry eye syndrome. This potentially damaging condition needs to be treated aggressively with lubrication and night taping to keep the lids closed as far as possible. Advise your surgeon if you experience prolonged dry eye symptoms.

If drooping of the lower lids occurs after surgery, which is rare, you will need to vigorously push the lid upward with your index finger across the lid every hour. Squeezing your eyes closed tightly can also help this condition by forcing swelling out of the lid more rapidly. As a last resort, further surgery may be indicated.

If too much fat is removed during surgery, the area around the eye can have a dug-out look, like a cadaver. Some surgeons recommend pushing fat back into its original location around the eye during the procedure. They maintain that as fat is removed the eye sinks back, causing it to appear sunken, smaller, and, hence, elderly. Other surgeons inject fat or transpose fat pads into the tear trough area along the inside of the lower lid. They believe this gives a more youthful appearance.

### When All Is Said and Done

Eliminating sagging, superfluous skin and fatty tissue around the eyes presents a younger, more rested appearance. The alert and youthful appearance will last for ten to twenty years, and for many people these results last even longer.

## CHIN AUGMENTATION

Aesthetic chin augmentation is a surgical procedure to reshape or increase the size of the chin for better projection and appearance. It can balance a profile by extending the chin in relationship to the nose. Patients with a relatively normal dental bite but weak or receding chins are the best candidates for chin augmentation.

### The Procedure

There are two basic approaches to chin augmentation. In some cases, it may be best to move the chin bone forward. In this technique, called genioplasty, the surgeon makes an incision inside the mouth to gain access to the chin bone area. Using surgical instruments, a horizontal cut is made through the bone. The lower portion of the separated bone is then shifted forward and stabilized. Because surgery is performed through an internal incision, the patient has no visible scar.

When a modest degree of chin augmentation is required to provide contour, the surgeon may recommend a chin implant or prosthesis as an alternative. Often a chin implant is made of a solid type of silicone (not the jelly type that was at the center of controversy in the breast implant issue). Implants now include extensions that are more anatomically natural.

With this technique, an incision is made either inside the mouth or externally on the underside of the chin. Working through the incision, the surgeon creates a pocket above the chin bone and under the muscles to insert an appropriately sized chin implant. The key to the surgery is to make a precise pocket. The scar from an external incision, made in the chin crease, is negligible.

I definitely prefer to approach the surgical site from the underside of the chin with an external incision, avoiding the muscles that run between the inside of the mouth and the edge of the chin. It is remotely possible to detach the chin muscles from the bone through the inside oral approach, and this is extremely difficult to correct. However, both approaches are certainly acceptable. The main consideration is your surgeon's comfort level with the preferred technique.

A chin implant is done along with nasal surgery perhaps 10 percent of the time, because a recessive chin accentuates a large nose. If facial balance is established, a proportional chin automatically gives the illusion that the nose is smaller.

### After Surgery

Some soreness and discomfort, which is easily controlled by pain medication, will occur after surgery. I advise a liquid diet for a week. Patients usually are up and around the same day and may go back to work with normal activities within a day or two if they do not object to wearing the dressings and chin strap in public. I have patients keep the Steri-Strip adhesive skin closures used in this procedure on for about one week. It is normal to feel a little depressed after any surgical procedure. This should pass in a few days.

### Risks and Limitations

Risks can include infection, bone reabsorption, chin numbness, displacement, extrusion, asymmetry, and bleeding. As always, the patient may be dissatisfied and surgery to revise the procedure may be needed.

I have had several implants migrate toward the mouth, and the patients could feel them with their tongues or when chewing. I corrected this by reentering the pockets and lowering the implants. I now suture through the implant and the lining of the bone to keep it in a more stable position.

Another potential problem is chin drop, or "witch's chin." The fleshy chin pad we all have is attached directly to the chin bone. If these attachments are interrupted by surgery, then the chin tissue could droop downward. This rare deformity only occurs when the original implant is placed through the mouth.

## SURGICAL LIP AUGMENTATION

Surgical procedures can offer a permanent alternative to collagen injections to augment the lips. This can be done using either surgical manipulation or grafts.

### The Procedure

*Grafts:* Grafts to enlarge the lips may be made up of skin, fat, or a combination of both. Grafts may come from the patient's body or from another donor. So far studies haven't found any significant difference between the two, although in my experience a patient's own skin is more permanent.

A graft taken from the patient's own body is called an autograft. An allograft is any human tissue that is transplanted from one body, usually a cadaver, to another. Treated pig's tissue, called a xenograft, may also be used.

The outer layer of any skin used is removed so that it doesn't form cysts. The tissue is then placed in the lip area. The graft material acts as a framework, like a trellis on which a vine grows. The vine is your own body tissue filling in and finally dissolving the artificial matrix.

Using processed skin from a donor saves a surgical step and avoids an incision that will leave a scar where the skin was harvested. However, if skin or muscle is available, say from a tummy or eyelid tuck, this can be used without an extra surgical step. It is also possible to augment the lip by placing synthetic material in the area rather than using donor skin. However, many surgeons have noted irregularities and protrusions under the skin.

***Surgical Augmentation:*** Another way to augment the lip is to move tissue from inside the mouth forward in a W pattern. This shifts mucosa toward the outside of the lip and rolls the lip outward, making it fuller in appearance. Problems with this method include asymmetries if one side of the mouth has more mucosal bulk than the other or because of healing problems. If the tissue is brought a little too far forward, rather than bulking up the lip itself, you can end up with a "monkey lip profile." This procedure also involves a good deal of healing time. The lip is quite stiff and sore for approximately three months. I find that this procedure works very well for my patients, but the long healing time and scars are a big downside.

### When All Is Said and Done

Lip enlargement may not be permanent, and this is one reason for the multitude of approaches. Cosmetic tattooing may also afford you the illusion of larger lips, and I recommend this procedure to many prospective patients. When I am doing the procedure, I favor using the patient's own skin, but if that is not an option, then my second choice is fat injection.

### FAT INJECTION

Fat injection, also called lipostructure infiltration, lipotransfer, and an assortment of other names, is a procedure that uses the patient's own body fat to fill in folds and wrinkles. It involves harvesting fat from one body area—usually the hip or tummy—and replacing it elsewhere, most commonly in the facial areas, especially cheek folds and lips.

The procedure is generally done under intravenous sedation or general anesthesia, and takes about an hour. It can be combined with other surgeries, and involves very little pain. The major problem with fat injection is that the body absorbs some of the fat. I tell patients there is a 50 percent chance that about 50 percent of the fat will be absorbed in a year. Transplanted fat is especially prone to reabsorption in areas of motion, as in the lips. Further injections may be necessary and can be repeated every six to twelve months.

Fat injection makes perfect sense as a rejuvenation procedure. We lose fat in our faces as we age, and we usually gain it elsewhere! An analysis of photos of people from high school through their 50th wedding anniversary using computerized morphing techniques (in a study by Dr. Val Lambros) clearly shows the loss of facial fat. The fat drops into the cheek, leaving a hollow tear trough below the eyes. The cheeks and lips lose their fullness, the temples thin, and the whole face narrows. If I were forced to pick only one single surgical procedure to rejuvenate someone's face, my first choice would be lipotransfer.

### Risks and Limitations

Bleeding, infection, scarring, numbness, donor site problems, contour irregularities, and fullness are some of the risks of this procedure. The biggest downside is that a patient's body may reabsorb the fat, thus undoing the gains. Be prepared to possibly have this procedure done more than once.

## OTOPLASTY, OR COSMETIC EAR SURGERY

The ear is 95 percent grown by the time a child is seven or eight years old. Many children suffer psychological damage from being teased because of their ears. Girls generally have it easier because they can hide their ears under their hair.

*"I was always self-conscious about the way my ears protruded,"* one patient told me. *"I was often teased and hardly ever wore my hair up. My family always reassured me I looked fine and that nobody ever notices ears anyway. It was little comfort, but at the time I was unaware that there was a procedure that could correct this."*

Otoplasty for a congenital cup ear deformity can be done before children begin school to minimize the amount of teasing they might get from classmates. The self-confidence gained from a one-hour procedure is certainly preferable to the hours and hours of counseling some of my young patients have had. It is very rewarding to see the newfound self-confidence when these youngsters return for postoperative visits and pictures.

Occasionally medical insurance companies will cover otoplasty if the patient has difficulty wearing a helmet, a hat, or athletic equipment. They may also take into consideration the discomfort of a patient awakened during the night by the ear rubbing on a pillow. I take a photo and send a letter of prior authorization to my patient's insurance company with a plea for help. This works about half of the time.

In adults, otoplasty is an out-of-pocket cosmetic procedure. Surgery is done on a same-day basis with very little postoperative pain or discomfort.

### Risks

Bleeding, infection, scarring, numbness, asymmetry, loss of cartilage, and bruising can occur. The original problem may recur if the cartilage memory is so strong it pushes the ear out again, in which case touch up surgery may be necessary.

### CHEEK IMPLANTS

Cheek implant surgery is fairly uncommon, comprising only 0.5 percent of the procedures done by physicians in the ASAPS. A cheek implant involves placing a prosthesis to give the patient a higher cheekbone. The approach can be through the mouth or through an incision made in each lower eyelid.

It's very hard to meet patient expectations with cheek implants. Patients often complain that the implants are too big or too small. Asymmetries are another common problem. This can happen because the implants have shifted, the natural structure of the cheekbones was different to begin with, or the implant was not placed precisely to the 10th of a millimeter from the midline on each side. I have also seen several infections from cheek implants.

I don't place cheek implants. Too many unhappy patients of other surgeons have dissuaded me from using the technique. If you are thinking about getting cheek implants, find a reputable surgeon with a lot of experience and a sharp artistic eye. One of my colleagues, a national authority on cheek implants who has a practice in California, has very few problems with implants. He has developed very specific ways to do the procedure and has superb results. Once you find a surgeon you are comfortable with, be sure to bring in photos that show the kind of results you hope to see so you and your doctor are clear about your expectations.

## SURFACE WORK

In addition to surgical procedures, there are a number of other options for enhancing your appearance. Many of them are simpler and less expensive than surgery, and require less recovery time. Of course there is always a trade-off, since many are also temporary. I don't perform these procedures myself, but my office staff or I will be happy to give you a referral to a local cosmetic care center or a colleague.

## BOTOX INJECTIONS

Botox is an extract of botulinum, a deadly poison that causes muscle paralysis. This is used to advantage in cosmetic surgery by carefully injecting the facial muscles to diminish wrinkling around the eyes when smiling and to ease furrowing of the brow. This procedure really works, but unfortunately it is temporary.

Some people believe resistance can be developed to the Botox injections, so subsequent injections last for shorter periods of time. It can be overdone or done inappropriately, so be certain your practitioner has plenty of experience in this area. A treatment generally lasts six months.

In the future, I expect Botox injections will be designed with a modified molecule that isn't detoxified by the body, so the results of the injections would be permanent. Patients could try the short-acting injection and if they like the results, commit to the permanent treatment.

## CHEMICAL PEELS

Chemical peels can be used to rejuvenate facial skin or to smooth facial wrinkles. Some of the results are truly amazing, but you need to be clear about what kind of peel you want, and be sure to find an experienced practitioner. Chemical peels can be mild, moderate, or strong.

### Mild Peels

The mild peel is what is known as a "lunch-hour" peel. A glycolic or salicylic acid solution is combined with dry ice to remove the outer layer of the epidermis. Patients are also started on a guided skin care program they carry out at home. It freshens and smoothes the skin and must be repeated frequently.

### Moderate Peels

The next step up is a moderate depth peel, what I call the "class reunion" peel. This peel gives the face a healthy, rosy glow and is a surefire bet to impress your friends without much expense or healing time. A chemical solution is applied to the skin with a sponge or cotton swab. Clinical judgment and a careful assessment of color changes on the skin allow the operator to judge the depth of the peel. This peel looks good right away and lasts about thirty days. It is extremely popular.

### Stronger Stuff

A strong peel consists of phenol or various mixtures of buffered phenol solutions. It is generally used to soften wrinkles. Strong peels have the potential to lighten the skin because the procedure affects the color cells or melanocytes within the skin's dermis, causing a porcelain or "tea-cup" appearance.

## TISSUE FILLERS AND COLLAGEN INJECTIONS

Hyaluronic acid fillers are injected to plump the tissue. Hyaluronic acid is cross-linked from either animal sources (rooster combs) or from bacterial fermentation sources. The cross-links resist absorption and prolong the filler effect.

Collagen, on the other hand, is protein derived from the connective tissue of cow or human skin, possibly the patient's own skin. Fillers are injected into the facial area to improve fine lines, major wrinkles, cheek folds, or for lip enlargement. The effects of these injections are temporary because the body absorbs them. The rate of absorption can vary, but the results usually last about six to twelve months, and less in areas of motion like the lips. There are myriad filler products now on the market, and the manufacturer's literature often seems to claim that their products last longer than we are actually seeing in practice.

Occasionally patients experience an unusually rapid reabsorption of the material. My first lip augmentation with collagen was done on a physician's wife. Her body absorbed all the collagen in two weeks. The injection cost $300. We were all ready to "go after that cow," and I no longer do collagen injections.

A lot of research is being done in this area. I expect permanent injectable compounds that can be placed in deeper facial wrinkles and cause no allergic reactions will be available in the future. Hyaluronic acid fillers are now the most popular fillers used in the U.S. and have supplanted collagen.

**Risks**

Three percent of people have a natural allergy to bovine (cow) collagen. All patients need to undergo a skin test before actual injections. An alternative is to take a portion of the patient's own skin and have this processed and injected. This avoids allergic reactions, but the reabsorption rate has been found to be somewhat faster than with bovine collagen. Newer products, like hyaluronic acid fillers, do not contain bovine collagen and don't require a skin test.

I've had some patients who had terrible soft tissue reactions and developed prolonged swelling that generally lasted over a year from an injection of collagen. The new tissue fillers are generally non-allergenic and more permanent so this procedure has improved significantly. Hopefully, in the future we will have injectable tissue-mimetic materials from customized human protein biomatrix fashioned from collagen-elastin to act as a permanent tissue filler which supports cell growth.

## LASER SKIN RESURFACING

Laser skin resurfacing involves applying the beam of a laser to the skin to alleviate wrinkles, acne or general scarring, age or brown spots, or sun-damaged skin. The procedure can produce great results, but it isn't for everybody. Darker-skinned patients may develop very dark areas following a laser procedure. People with lighter complexions and blue eyes tend to do very well.

The best results are achieved with a full-face laser procedure because this uniformly stretches the skin throughout the facial area and produces a more homogeneous color. Laser resurfacing can produce dramatic and pronounced skin tightening when the entire face is resurfaced. This impressive improvement results from rearrangement of the collagen bundles as the skin shrinks. This is why some people refer to laser resurfacing as a laser facelift.

In preparing for a laser procedure, patients must stop taking the oral acne medication, Accutane, for at least one year because it impairs healing. A history of cold sores indicates that a patient may need to use prophylactic antibiotics to fight the herpes virus, which may be activated by the laser treatment.

### Everything You Wanted to Know About Lasers but Were Afraid to Ask

Do you know where the word laser comes from? In spite of watching all those *Star Wars* movies, neither did I. It's really an acronym for Light Amplification by Stimulated Emission of Radiation. An element—often carbon dioxide or erbium—is stimulated to emit radiation that is applied to the skin. Varied wavelengths are applied for a multitude of skin conditions.

Laser light is different from normal light in that it travels in a single direction even over long distances. Ordinary light spreads out and is not focused. More power can be produced with a laser than by any other light source, even the sun.

### Laser-Tissue Interaction

A laser beam interacts with human tissue in several different ways. As the light first strikes the skin, a small fraction is reflected from the surface. The remainder of the light goes into the tissue and is reflected from cell walls, nuclei, and connective fibers. The energy is absorbed by the tissue and heats it. This produces the laser's major clinical effect.

### After Surgery

I used to describe in detail how scary a patient's face would look the first week after laser treatment. No matter how hard I tried to communicate this to patients, they invariably said, "You never told me it would look this bad!" So I asked some of my patients for permission to take pictures of them postoperatively, and I now show prospective patients how they will probably look on each postoperative day. This allows patients who decide to go ahead with the procedure to be clearly informed. It allows others to leave my clinic firmly resolved never to consider laser treatments again.

In an average treatment, crusts will form on the skin. Those from the erbium laser will heal in about five to seven days. With the carbon dioxide laser, healing takes about 10 days. The face may be red for a month after the erbium laser treatment and for several months after carbon dioxide. In both cases the redness will fade over the subsequent year. Avoiding all sun exposure and using sunscreen is imperative after a laser procedure to avoid permanent patchy color changes.

**Risks**

Possible risks include infection, herpes outbreaks, postoperative scarring, permanent color changes to the skin, prolonged redness or itching, permanent patchy spots due to sun exposure, and failure of the surgery. Specific safety precautions to protect the patient's eyes and teeth are imperative. Make certain that a designated laser safety officer (LSO) has inspected and approved the facility at which the procedure will take place.

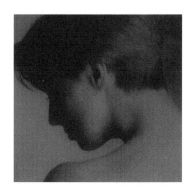

*chapter 8*

# BODY WORK

"Plastic surgeons consider themselves sculptors.

Nowhere else is the oft-used term 'body sculpting'

more applicable. Using living tissue, plastic surgery artists

can shape, mold, and form the human body."

– Anonymous

## ABDOMINOPLASTY OR TUMMY TUCK

Abdominoplasty, commonly called a tummy tuck, is a procedure designed to tighten sagging abdominal muscles and give the stomach area a flatter and smoother appearance. The procedure is most commonly done on women after they have had children. Many women are simply restoring their past figures from B.C. (Before Children). This isn't vanity; it's a reclaiming of self, or a healthy undoing of the past. Pregnancy can cause the lower abdominal muscles to stretch out and displace from the midline, and excess subcutaneous tissue may accumulate. The lower abdomen is often a fat storage area in women, probably designed by nature to protect them from famine. It's like the hump on a camel and is extremely resistant to diet and exercise. Exercise will strengthen and firm the muscles, but all the sit-ups in the world won't bring them back if your abdominal muscles have spread apart due to pregnancy.

Only four percent of patients undergoing tummy tucks are men, and most patients are of baby boomer age. Abdominoplasty can flatten a protruding abdomen, but the trade-off is a scar running along the lower abdomen. This sometimes can be limited by endoscopic surgery. Additional scars may be around the belly button, and some may extend from hip to hip, depending on how much skin has to be removed. The scars are permanent.

Abdominoplasty is not a weight-loss procedure. It benefits patients who are in relatively good shape but are plagued by an extensive fat deposit or loose abdominal skin unresponsive to diet or exercise. Some older patients who have lost skin elasticity and developed mild areas of fullness can also be helped.

Some patients store fat inside the abdomen around the intestines. They look like they have a beer belly, but there isn't really a large amount of fat on the outer abdominal wall. These patients aren't candidates for abdominoplasty. The large amount of inside tummy fat pushes out the entire abdominal wall. This overall protrusion can't be corrected surgically because the muscles are stretched everywhere rather than simply separated in the middle, as is usually the case following pregnancies.

If you plan to lose weight, do your best to do so before abdominoplasty. Surgeons can obtain flatter results by removing as much skin as possible. Women who plan on a future pregnancy should wait to have abdominoplasty because the vertical muscles running up and down the abdomen—that six-pack we hear so much about—will stretch during pregnancy, undoing surgical repairs. If someone is undecided about having a baby in the future or isn't planning on a family for many years, I let them decide if the surgery is worth it. In general, plastic surgeons defer abdominoplasty until after a woman has finished with child bearing.

This is not a simple operation. Your surgeon will want to take a health history, and determine the extent of fat deposits, and your skin and muscle tone. Be sure to tell your surgeon if you smoke, and report all medications and supplements you are taking. I will not operate on active smokers.

Tell your surgeon what changes to your appearance you expect to see. Based on your exam and a discussion with your surgeon, you may decide not to have the surgery at all. Ask your surgeon for a candid response about limitations based on your personal anatomy. Maybe liposuction alone could achieve a good result. Balance your expectations with a realistic goal. Review photos of prior patients with a preoperative anatomy similar to yours and compare their outcomes with what you want to see.

Regardless of which variation of abdominoplasty you and your surgeon choose, be certain the most revealing clothing you are likely to wear will cover the incision lines. **It's a good idea to wear a swimsuit the morning of surgery to use as a reference. I draw the incisions for my patients while they're looking in a mirror, so they can verify their satisfaction with the incision placement.**

*"Belly be gone,"* exclaimed one of my patients as she pretended to cast a spell on her tummy while looking in the mirror.

### The Procedure

Abdominoplasty is usually done as same-day surgery. Generally, surgeons do abdominoplasty under general anesthesia, so you'll be completely asleep with a breathing tube. Other surgeons, depending on the extent of the procedure, choose local anesthesia with heavy intravenous sedation to keep you in a twilight sleep. You shouldn't feel any pain but possibly could feel some pressure or tugging.

## TYPES OF ABDOMINOPLASTY

There are several different abdominoplasty procedures used, depending on the patient's needs and anatomy. Discuss the procedure carefully with your surgeon to determine which one is right for you.

### Endoscopic Abdominoplasty

Endoscopic abdominoplasty is used in the rare cases where someone suffers from muscle relaxation but has good skin tone and needs little or no skin removed. In general, all abdominoplasties will begin with liposuction to smooth out unwanted fullness in certain areas. Then a one- to two-inch incision is made in a skin crease or an old surgical scar. The skin is elevated along the middle of the abdomen, sometimes all the way up to the lower end of the breastbone. Special endoscopy instruments are used to place strong muscle sutures to flatten the middle of your abdomen. Additional small incisions may be made higher on your abdomen. The procedure lasts about two hours.

### Modified or Limited Abdominoplasty

If a modified or limited tummy-tuck is indicated, following liposuction, the lower abdominal muscles on either side of the abdomen will be exposed through a crosswise incision along the upper pubic hairline. Incision length depends on your anatomy. Sutures will be placed in the midline to tighten your tummy. Additional sutures may be placed on the sides of your lower abdomen to tighten these areas.

Excess skin and some underlying fatty tissue are trimmed. Finally, additional liposuction contouring may be done before your incision is closed. A drainage tube usually is placed to prevent any accumulation of blood or serum during the first few days after surgery. This procedure usually lasts between one and a half to two and a half hours.

### Complete or Classic Abdominoplasty

Complete abdominoplasty generally requires an incision from hip to hip across the lower abdomen. The actual length of the incision depends on your anatomy. Your natural belly-button should be left attached to the underlying muscles. Abdominal muscles are tightened by pulling them into your midline and stitching them where they used to be. This firms up the abdominal wall. Additional sutures can be placed to narrow the waistline.

Skin and subcutaneous tissue are stretched and removed. A new opening is made for your navel through the overlying skin. One or two suction drains will be placed prior to suture closure. Usually butterfly skin tapes, sterile dressings, and an abdominal binder are applied. The surgery may last two to three hours. I always use compression boots during the procedure and into the recovery room to squeeze blood through the legs to prevent blood clots from forming.

### After Surgery

Someone will need to drive you home when you are discharged and be around the house to help you for a few days. Pain from a full tummy-tuck can be about eight on a scale of one to 10, with 10 being a kidney stone and nine the delivery of a baby. Usually the abdomen is bruised for about three weeks and feels kind of numb and funny for several months, and in some cases to a slight degree for the rest of the patient's life. This is not disabling, but the area doesn't feel "quite right" when touched.

You will be discharged several hours after the procedure is done. You will have one or two drains. A drain is a small plastic tube connected to a light bulb shaped reservoir. The compressible reservoir creates gentle suction to remove excess fluid from the surgical area. The recovery room nurse will teach you how to care for the drain prior to your discharge from the surgery center. You'll receive pain pills and, possibly, a prophylactic antibiotic. I prefer to have my complete tummy tuck patients go home with bladder catheters, so they don't have to get out of bed during the night to urinate. My patients wear elastic stockings to help prevent blood clots in the legs.

### Road to Recovery

After an abdominoplasty you will need to avoid heavy lifting or vigorous exercise for six to eight weeks, so there is definitely a prolonged recovery period. Don't try to lift anything heavier than about 10 pounds (the equivalent of a full grocery bag) during this time. Carefully lifting your children should be all right as long as you hold them close to yourself. Think of the operation as a hernia repair from "stem to stern," and treat yourself gently.

I ask patients to walk hunched over for about a week to keep tension off the incision line. You can return to work in a week or two, if your job doesn't involve heavy lifting. If you have a physically demanding job, you may need to return on light duty for a month. It may take a month or two before you feel like your old self. Studies show people who are in the best shape possible before surgery have the fastest recovery.

The incision will be pink for several months and then fade over the subsequent year. If your scar rises, becomes tender, or stays reddened, you may need additional treatment such as a cortisone injection. Mild depression is normal after surgery. It is a result of biochemical changes caused by the anesthesia and surgery, and should go away fairly quickly.

## Risks and Complications

The problems I've had with tummy-tuck surgery tend to be the same as those for all cosmetic surgical procedures. Irregularity or asymmetry may persist, and touch-up surgery may be required. A number of patients develop fluid collections after their drains are removed. Sometimes this requires draining, which is done with a needle in the clinic. Rare instances of permanent fluid build-up have been reported. Treatment involves another operation to remove the tissue lining that is continuing to form abnormal fluid.

Bad scarring is another possible complication. Infection is rare and usually is treated with antibiotics or surgical drainage. Excessive bleeding is unusual, and the drainage tubes are there to handle this. Geometrical problems like elevation of the pubic hairline or lack of central placement of the belly-button are potential risks. I curve the incision over the pubis and make precise preoperative measurements to prevent this from occurring.

Blood clots can be avoided by being active after your procedure. I use compressive stockings or mechanical devices on the operating table to squeeze the patient's calves. Walking as soon as possible is helpful to maintain muscle strength and prevent blood clots. Surgeons may instruct patients to do ankle and foot exercises to improve blood circulation.

Smoking can cause serious complications, and smokers can suffer skin loss. See the section on facelifts for more details.

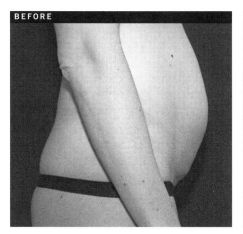
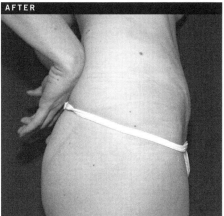

Abdominoplasty to undo muscle laxity from pregnancy

### When All Is Said and Done

Abdominoplasty won't give you the perfect washboard abdomen you had as a teenager, but it will improve your appearance to a great degree. Results are long lasting, especially if you stay on a healthy diet and exercise program. There will be permanent scars.

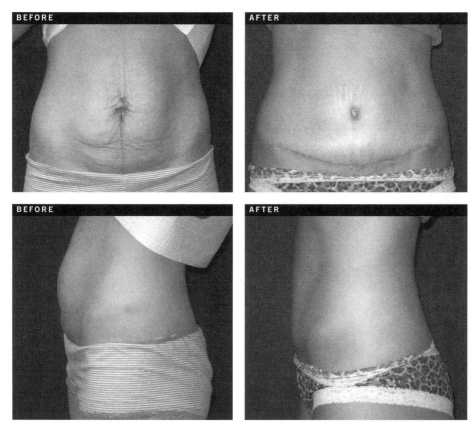

Abdominoplasty (front and left side) showing the incision six weeks postop to refine entire abdomen

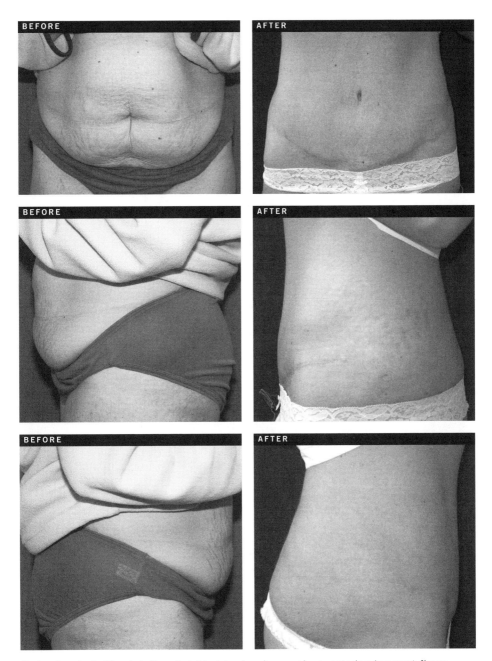

Abdominoplasty (front, left and right side views) — patient restoring her past figure from B.C. (Before Children)

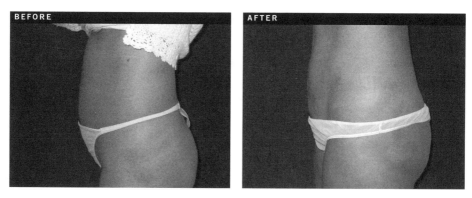

Abdominoplasty (tummy tuck) for muscle relaxation

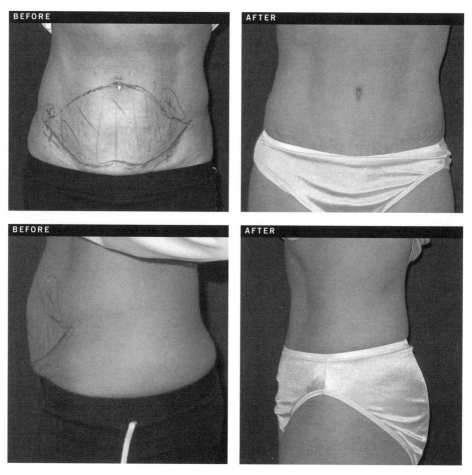

Preoperative markings showing the extensive amount of skin removal from the belly button down to the pubis in a complete or classic abdominoplasty (tummy tuck)

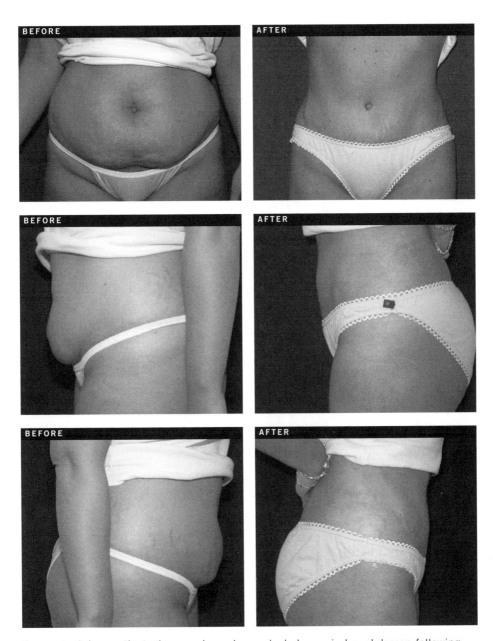

Tummy tuck in a patient who experienced a marked change in her abdomen following the birth of her first child

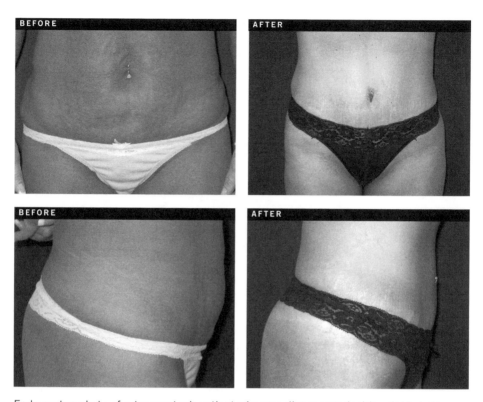

Early postop photo of a tummy tuck patient who was disconcerted with wrinkled skin above her belly button (umbilicus)

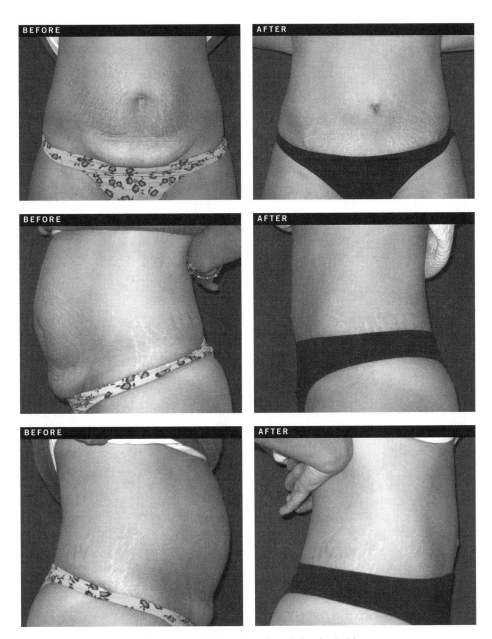

Tummy tuck demonstrating removal of overhanging abdominal skin

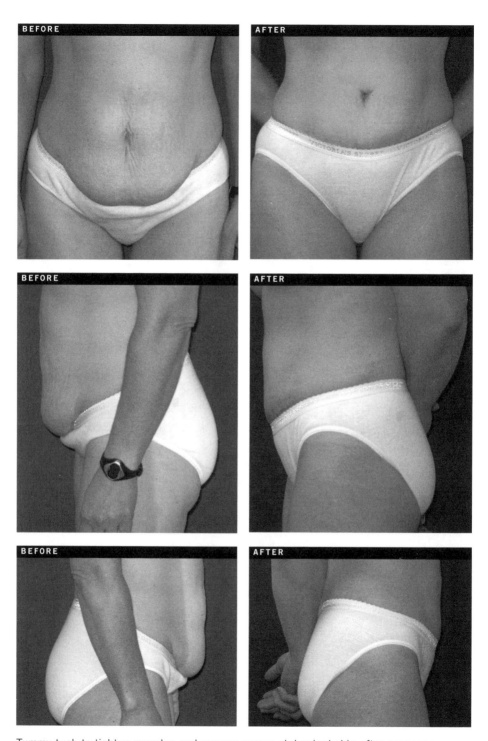

Tummy tuck to tighten muscles and remove excess abdominal skin after pregnancy

## BUTTOCKS LIFT

Buttocks lifts are fairly uncommon, comprising less than one percent of surgical and nonsurgical cosmetic procedures. Either from aging, weight loss, or just plain genetics, in some people the ligaments supporting the buttocks relax. A procedure has been devised to remove a crescent of tissue from the uppermost aspect of each buttock, while the bottom portion of the buttock is elevated. The procedure is usually accompanied by some liposuction. In some cases the incisions can be extended all the way around to the front of the body and combined with a tummy tuck for a 360-degree truncoplasty.

Correct surgical technique involves a detailed knowledge of anatomy so that the supporting tissue layers, called the fascial systems, can be exactly positioned to enhance the long-term success of the procedure. Cosmetic surgeons attending national meetings are reporting many more requests for buttocks augmentation. Courses have been organized to educate members about this increasingly popular procedure.

If you are considering a buttocks lift or augmentation, ask your surgeon for photos of previous patients and, if possible, discuss the surgery with one of them. This procedure involves a lengthy incision with a good deal of scarring, although the scar can usually be hidden within the bikini line.

### Risks

The most common risks include bad scarring, infection, bleeding, numbness, patient dissatisfaction, the need for possible revisional surgery, and recurrence of sagging over time.

## LIPOSUCTION

Liposuction is the most common surgical procedure performed by American Board of Plastic Surgery members. Liposuction removes deposits of subcutaneous fat over diverse areas of the body—including the face and neck, upper arms, trunk, abdomen, hips, buttocks, inner and outer thighs, knees, and occasionally the calves and ankles. Some of these areas are resistant to diet and exercise, and many scientists believe they were designed by nature to function as fat storage regions meant to withstand famine. Some studies claim these subcutaneous cells appear different from the fat cells in other areas of the body under microscopic analysis.

*"I decided to have liposuction done to my saddlebag areas, inner thighs, and love handles after years and years of exercising and weight training,"* one patient said. *"These areas never improved, no matter what I did."*

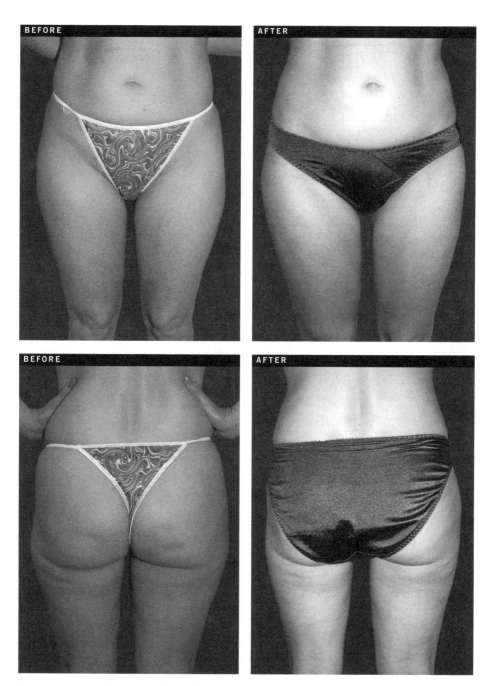

Suction assisted lipectomy (fat suction) of the inside and outside thighs, hips and buttocks: note the rippling and waviness present on the backside preoperatively

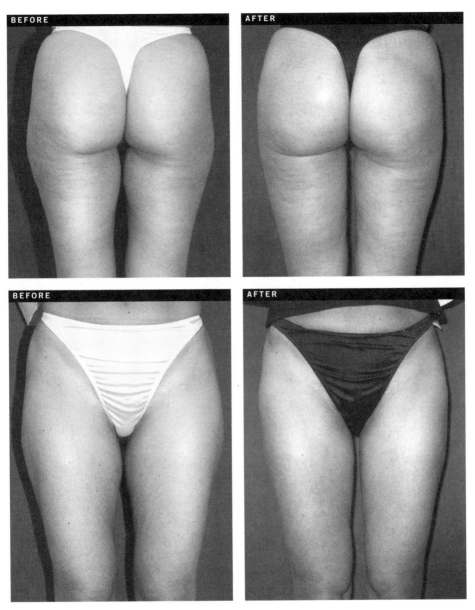

Liposuction (back and front views) to reduce localized subcutaneous fullness over buttocks, inner and outer thighs

A person is born with only so many fat cells, as they are born with only so many muscle cells. These cells grow and shrink when you gain and lose weight, but they don't change in number. And unlike some of the tissues in your body, fat does not regenerate. That's what makes liposuction such an attractive surgery: the results, at least in the suctioned area, are permanent. If you subsequently gain weight it may settle in the remaining fat cells in a suctioned area, but it will never have the same bulk as it did before the surgery. The fat cells simply aren't there anymore.

The best candidates for liposuction are people of normal weight who have excellent overlying skin tone, who have localized areas of fullness, and who realize liposuction is not a weight loss procedure. Age is of less importance when it comes to liposuction, but older patients may not have the same skin elasticity as younger people. The popular literature in the mid-1980s stated that anyone over 40 years old couldn't have liposuction, but the age has been raised. I've done liposuction on a 63-year-old woman with a surprisingly good result.

Liposuction is as much art as science, and it is important to choose a surgeon you feel comfortable with and have confidence in. When you come in for an initial consultation with me, you should expect to spend a couple of hours in my office. I show prospective patients a video describing the proce-dure, and give them a book of before and after photos and patient testimonials so they can get an idea of my work and the results that are possible. Then I examine the patient, in the presence of a nurse, and we discuss together the results the patient would like to see and the best way to achieve them.

It is vital that you be as clear as possible about your expectations. If you are hoping for a perfectly flat stomach, for example, it might take a tummy tuck as well as liposuction to achieve the results you want. Sometimes it is better to do a little more than just the areas you are concerned about to achieve a smooth long-term result. If you store a lot of fat in your hips and stomach, for example, suctioning only the hips can leave you looking perpetually pregnant if you later gain weight. Your doctor can advise you about the best way to achieve the look you want. Liposuction can have excellent results:

*"I am elated with my new figure. I'm eight pounds lighter and two sizes smaller,"* one patient said. *"I went out in public in a swimsuit for the first time since I was a teenager,"* another told me. *"I was always self-conscious about my big saddlebags. Since my surgery, I feel like I look normal for the first time in years. I can wear pants again without looking bottom heavy, and my legs don't ache when I stand up for more than an hour. That's good, since I'm two sizes smaller now and you have to stand up a lot when you're trying on new clothes."*

Depending on your original body shape, your results may be more subtle.

*"I really noticed a difference in the size of my legs,"* one woman said. *"They looked long and lean. When I put on my jeans they fit so much better. My body shape from the waist down was more appealing."*

If your expectations were realistic, you should be pleased with your result, no matter how subtle or dramatic.

Liposuction is often performed with associated surgeries, such as a facelift following suction of the neck area, a tummy tuck following suction of the abdominal wall, or a thigh lift following suction of the area to be tightened.

**The Procedure**

Several different liposuction techniques, including tumescent, super-wet, power-assisted, and ultrasound-assisted lipoplasty, may be used. Your doctor will go over each of them and determine which is best for your particular case.

Liposuction is generally done on a same-day basis, often in a surgical center specializing in cosmetic surgery. High volume procedures, in which more than eleven pounds of fluid will be removed, should be done at a hospital. High volume procedures carry much higher risks, and I generally don't recommend them.

You will meet with your doctor before the surgery, and the areas to be suctioned will be marked with a felt-tip marker to ensure accuracy during surgery and to make sure the patient and doctor are on the same wavelength. This is where you need to be very clear about your expectations. If you are having your buttocks suctioned, do you want them to be full and rounded or flat and boyish? Unless you tell your surgeon what your own idea of beauty is, you'll end up with his or hers.

Once you are marked, the surgery will begin. A narrow tube called a cannula is attached to a vacuum machine and passed through small skin incisions, which are strategically placed in skin folds whenever possible. By a repetitive gliding and suction motion, tissue is removed and sculpted until good contour and symmetry is established. It's a fairly common practice to inject a wetting solution into the surgical area prior to beginning the suction. This enhances results and greatly diminishes blood loss. Using a wetting solution is fairly standard practice and allows a dilute local anesthetic and adrenaline to be deposited. This can diminish discomfort during the procedure and decrease postoperative bruising.

During liposuction, fat isn't the only thing being removed. Vital body fluids are being removed as well, so it's important to replace these fluids to prevent shock. You'll be carefully monitored during the procedure and will receive intravenous fluids during and immediately after surgery.

## ULTRASOUND-ASSISTED LIPOSUCTION (UAL)

Although the development of suction-assisted lipectomy has advanced the field of plastic surgery, specific areas were until recently not as amenable to treatment, such as fibrous areas on the back, the breast area in men, and revisional liposuction in some patients. It was discovered that ultrasound energy delivered through a hollow titanium probe into the subcutaneous tissue could selectively destroy fat cells. Usually this procedure is followed by traditional liposuction to remove remaining liquefied material not harvested by the ultrasound probe. Some patients also see a dramatic tightening of the skin.

There are some additional risks to using UAL compared to traditional liposuction, including skin burns and micro-fragmentation of the cannula. Since this is a newer procedure, there may be additional risks that are not yet evident. I have seen some skin irregularities develop during the procedure, which generally resolve on their own. UAL is touted as having fewer postoperative problems such as bruising, but this has not really been a factor in my experience because the classic suction-assisted technique is always used following the UAL, and bruising is normal with this procedure.

Some plastic surgeons melt the underlying fat through the skin with an external ultrasound machine. This requires injecting fluid into the underlying tissue, so there will still be an incision or a puncture site. Only moderate amounts of fat can be removed with this technique and a large volume would have to be done at multiple surgical sessions. As of now, the best bet for removing larger volumes still involves surgery.

### Anesthesia

Your procedure will be done under local, regional, or general anesthesia. Discuss the various options with your surgeon to choose the one that is best for you.

***Local, with or without sedation***: If small amounts of fat or a limited number of body sites are involved, a local anesthetic can be used to numb the area. You may have a mild sedative to help you relax. This method is referred to as IV (intravenous) sedation or monitored anesthesia care (MAC).

*Regional*: For more extensive procedures a regional anesthetic can be used. This comes in the form of an epidural block. A catheter is inserted into the spine in a relatively painless procedure and a continuous flow of anesthetic is delivered that results in no feeling from the waist down. You're fully awake when this method is used. The same anesthesia is used in childbirth.

*General*: You may opt for general anesthesia if you are having a large amount of fat removed. In this case you will be unconscious throughout the procedure and may have a breathing tube and catheter inserted for the duration of the procedure.

## After Surgery

Most patients report that pain is three on a scale of one to 10, but some report seven or eight. Some fluid will drain from the incisions. You may experience pain, burning, swelling, bleeding, and numbness. You will be prescribed pain medication and anti-nausea medication, and can expect to feel stiff and sore for a few days. If you have any unusual symptoms not outlined on your discharge sheet, call your surgeon immediately.

To control swelling and to help your skin fit its new contours, you will have to wear a snug elastic surgical garment, like a girdle, for six weeks following your surgery. This is usually worn 24 hours a day for the first three weeks, and 12 hours a day, during the daytime, for the last three weeks.

Following this surgery, patients are sore but most feel better during the first week. Many patients compare the feeling to the muscle soreness you experience following a too-strenuous workout. You may experience some mild discomfort for several weeks. Swelling following the procedure may last up to six months, although many patients see a dramatic improvement within the first week.

Even though you may not want to do it, walking is the best way to speed up your recovery. It helps reduce swelling and prevents blood clots. If your ankles swell from walking, your body is telling you to cut down your activities and get off your feet more. Sit down, put your feet up, and flex your ankles frequently to help your circulation. Avoid strenuous activity for about two weeks.

Most people are able to return to work in about a week, but it may be as little as a few days, depending on your procedure and the kind of work you do. Stitches will dissolve in about ten days.

**Road to Recovery**

You may feel nervous or anxious in the days and weeks following your procedure. You may be stiffer and more sore than you had expected, or you may have thought you would look a lot different a lot sooner. Many patients feel somewhat depressed following surgery. This is a normal reaction to the stress your body has experienced and should go away in a few days. Be patient. The more time passes, the better you will look and feel.

Bruising will improve within about three weeks, but you may experience some residual swelling for as long as six months or even more. Don't expose your skin to the sun or a tanning booth while bruising is still present. This may fixate the blood cell pigment in the skin, and the bruising may become more prolonged or even permanent.

The areas of suction may feel numb and strange for a couple of months, but this should improve over time. Some areas may be tender to the touch for several months. The small scars from your incisions will fade gradually and should eventually either disappear altogether or become almost unnoticeable.

**Risks**

Your risks with this procedure are minimal if you are physically healthy and a good candidate for the surgery, and if your doctor is adequately trained. If you have heart or lung disease, diabetes, or poor blood circulation, liposuction carries some increased risks that should be discussed with your doctor.

Although complications are very rare, they do occur. Possible complications during the surgery can include excessive fluid loss, which can lead to shock. You will be given intravenous fluids during the procedure to prevent this. Rare but serious complications include friction burns, damage to the skin or nerves, perforation injuries to vital organs, and adverse reactions to injected fluids or anesthesia.

Post-surgical complications are similar to those of other surgeries, and can include infection, healing delays, blood clots, and fluid accumulation requiring drainage. Complications are rare when an experienced medical team performs the procedure in a licensed surgical facility.

Though serious medical complications from liposuction are rare, the risks increase if a greater number and size of areas are treated at one time. Removal of large volumes of fat and fluid may require sizeable volumes of preinjection fluid and longer operating times. The combination of these factors can create hazards for infections, delays in healing, improper fluid balance, shock, and unfavorable drug reactions.

The most common problems with liposuction are cosmetic. Your skin surface may be irregular, asymmetric, or even baggy, depending on your skin tone. Sometimes additional surgeries can improve these imperfections. Touch-up surgery is widespread following liposuction. Residual areas of fullness are quite common, and your surgeon may allow for a follow-up procedure in his fee. As always, you will still have to pay for any new surgical center charges.

**When All Is Said and Done**

If your expectations were realistic, you should be pleased with your results, no matter how subtle or dramatic. The effects of liposuction are permanent—once the fat cells are gone from an area, they won't come back. If you gain weight, it may still migrate to the remaining fat cells in your suctioned areas, or it may settle somewhere else. On the other hand, many patients lose even more weight following the procedure, probably because they feel and look better and are more likely to get out and exercise. There is little if any permanent scarring with this procedure.

## LOWER BODY LIFT

A lower body lift is a massive procedure and involves direct surgical excision of redundant skin and subcutaneous tissue in a patient who is not an appropriate candidate for liposuction alone. Lower body lifts are uncommon, accounting for only 0.5 percent of the work of American Society of Aesthetic Plastic Surgery members. Ninety-five percent of patients were women.

This procedure has many variations but generally involves a circumferential or near circumferential incision to remove excessive abdominal, waist, buttock, and thigh tissue. This may be an inpatient procedure, and patients must be in excellent physical health to be candidates. Patients having this procedure usually have lost significant amounts of weight, often after undergoing a stomach bypass procedure.

## THIGH LIFT

Prior to liposuction, thigh lifts were more frequent. Now thigh lifts are uncommon, making up less than one percent of American Society of Aesthetic Plastic Surgery members' work. The procedure is generally reserved for correcting skin laxity, and subcutaneous fat is suctioned rather than cut out. Ninety-eight percent of thigh lifts are done on women.

### The Procedure

Before surgery, the patient is marked while standing to verify the areas to be suctioned and the placement of the incision lines, which can usually be hidden in the groin crease. This procedure is always done under general anesthesia. Liposuction is done to remove excess fat and then a crescent of skin and subcutaneous tissue is excised. Specific firm, dense tissue planes are anatomically identified and sutures are placed in these firm layers to give adequate support to the inner thigh area.

### Risks and Complications

Complications are the same as those described for liposuction. In addition, scar migration may occur because it is difficult to excise the desired amount of skin without having the incision migrate up and backwards toward the buttock. After the surgery the patient must avoid vigorous activity for six weeks to let the dense connective tissue in this area heal completely.

Labial separation, early recurrence of sagging skin, and possible premature separation or opening of the surgical incision also can be complications of thigh lifts.

## UPPER ARM LIFT

Upper arm lifts aren't very common, comprising less than one percent of ASAPS members' procedures. I prefer to treat the upper arm area with liposuction and avoid excising skin and subcutaneous tissue if possible because of the noticeable scar involved. However, some patients may be candidates for skin excision if they don't mind the scar or don't intend to expose their arms much. Whenever possible, I confine the scar to the armpit area rather than carry it down the inside of the upper arm.

### The Procedure

Once liposuction is done, either a crescent or, depending on how much is removed, a goldfish-shaped area of tissue is removed. The wound then is closed. The risks are similar to those for liposuction and thigh lifts. In addition, upper arm numbness could be a problem. Sometimes the scar elevates, becomes firm, and stays pink or red. This condition is treated with cortisone injections until the scar's appearance improves. Any scar is permanent.

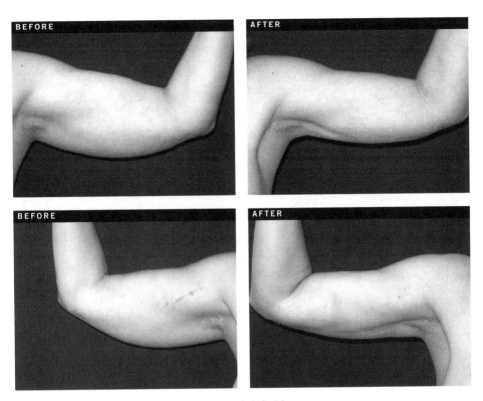

Liposuction to give the upper arms improved definition

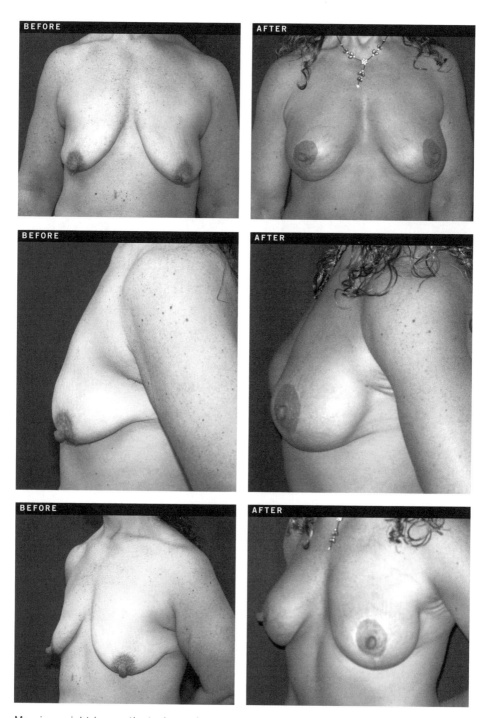

Massive weight loss patient who underwent a "total body lift" (upper and lower body lift) including: buttocks lift, thigh lift, truncoplasty, upper arm lift and breast lift with implants- over one year postop

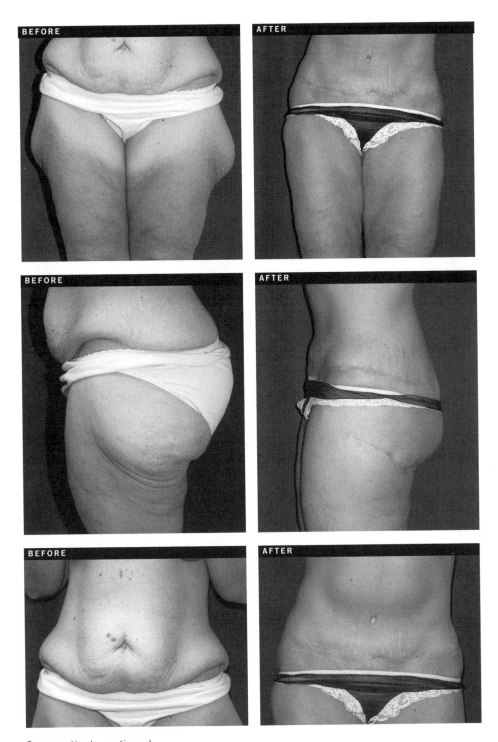

Same patient, continued

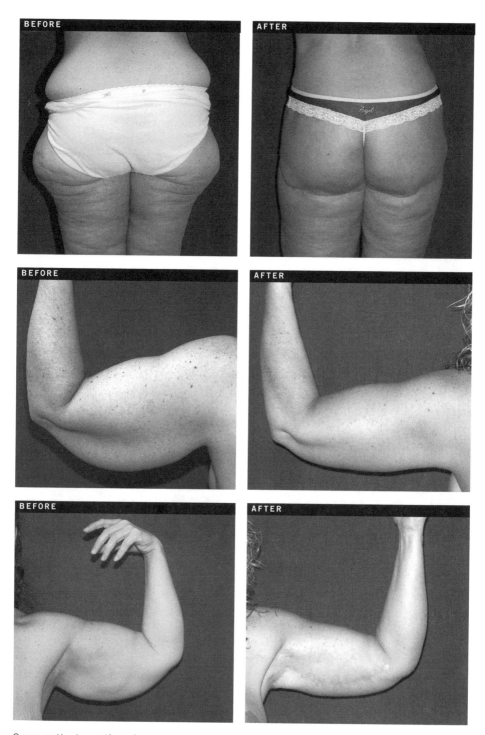

Same patient, continued

## WHAT'S ON THE HORIZON

### Hand Rejuvenation

Hand rejuvenation is an often-ignored area of cosmetic surgery. Aging hands may develop dark brown or tan sun or age spots. The tissue over the back of the hand may thin with grooves showing between tendons. Laser treatments can be used to remove dark spots and fat injections can plump the area and rejuvenate the back of the hand. A new cream used in treating skin cancer has also been found to rejuvenate sun-exposed skin on the backs of the hands.

### Vein Treatments

Sclerotherapy involves injecting a corrosive substance into the small blood vessels of the legs. This substance may be a dense solution of saline or an irritant. Laser treatment is a gentler, kinder way of treating face veins, but injections work better for the leg veins and are still the gold standard.

Larger veins are not amenable to sclerotherapy, and very large veins, such as varicose veins, must be surgically removed. Problems with sclerotherapy can include dark spots, permanent color changes, skin loss, especially in smokers, infection, and the necessity of repeating the procedure.

### CoolSculpting™ Treatments

CoolSculpting™ was developed by Harvard scientists. It is a FDA-cleared, patented procedure that uses a targeted cooling process to kill fat cells underneath the skin, literally freezing them to the point of elimination. Only the fat cells are frozen. CoolSculpting™ doesn't burn, shatter or extract any cells. Your healthy skin cells remain. Once crystallized, the fat cells die and are naturally eliminated from your body. Patients experience changes as quickly as three weeks after the treatment, and will experience the most dramatic results after two months. Your body continues to flush out fat cells four to six months after treatment. Unlike most other methods of fat reduction, CoolSculpting™ involves no needles, surgery, or downtime.

After a CoolSculpting™ treatment, you can typically get right back to your day. Each treatment lasts one hour. After one visit, you'll typically see a noticeable reduction of fat. After a few months, your clothes will fit better and you will look better, as long as you maintain your normal diet and exercise, your long-term results should remain stable.

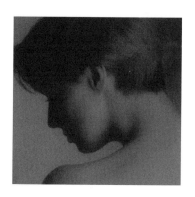

*chapter 9*

# PLASTIC SURGERY

# FOR MEN

"Why not do it? You have body work done on your car."

— Sylvester Stallone

*W*omen have plastic surgery much more often than men do. Men have 40 percent of all cosmetic ear surgery, or otoplasty, and 30 percent of rhinoplasty. About 20 percent of patients who undergo chemical peels are male, as are 15 percent who have eyelid tucks. Men have only 10 percent of facelifts and forehead lifts. Just four percent of tummy-tuck patients are male.

There is one area where men outnumber the women: Men receive 90 percent of hair transplants. And there is one category of cosmetic surgery that deals with men exclusively: the treatment of chest enlargement, or gynecomastia. But more men than ever are requesting cosmetic surgery. Men want to look young and fit.

In my practice, men request these procedures most often:
- Liposuction—most commonly for the neck, chin, jaw line, abdomen, love handles, and chest.
- Facial cosmetic surgery—eyelid tucks, facelifts, chin implants, and rhinoplasty.
- Hair techniques—either to remove excess hair, or to add more.
- Trunk surgery—tummy tucks can tighten saggy abdomens and waists.

There are definite differences in how procedures are performed on men and women. The following explains some of the most common procedures.

## BALDNESS

Incredible progress has been made in treating baldness. Re-establishing a hairline by rearranging the scalp hair pattern, using surgical flaps to rotate from the side of the head onto the front, is now commonplace. This is a larger surgery with more down time than hair transplantation. Some practitioners combine hair transplants with surgical flaps. I would recommend seeking a practitioner who has a special interest in baldness and microfollicular grafts. Many clinics specialize solely in these procedures.

You may have seen hair transplants done many years ago with that "corncob" or "cobblestone" look. Follicular unit hair transplantation using micrografting techniques avoids this effect. The hair follicle is the growth area of the hair. Follicular unit transplantation involves using a dissecting stereomicroscope to divide naturally occurring follicular units from a donor strip of hair. All this extra effort is definitely worth it, as the results are natural and youthful looking.

On the nonsurgical side, there is a lot of research going on to discover new treatments for baldness. Perhaps a medication will be found soon that really works quickly and definitively in virtually everyone, and is not exorbitantly priced.

## EYELID TUCK OR BLEPHAROPLASTY

The male upper eyelid is generally fuller than the female, and excess skin tends to appear more masculine. I'm always conservative in removing upper eyelid tissue on men. This fullness is associated in our culture with an appearance of strength and power. Removing too much tissue will feminize the upper lid.

## TREATING GYNECOMASTIA OR BREAST ENLARGEMENT

Gynecomastia is breast enlargement in men. This may come on in the early teenage years and can be extremely embarrassing. Unfortunately, most insurance companies have little sympathy for the psychological damage these young men can suffer. The condition often runs in families, and sometimes a guilt-ridden father will bring in his son, hoping for a better adolescence than he experienced. Gynecomastia can also be associated with the use of marijuana or with certain rare medical conditions. Overweight males make more estrogen, contributing to the problem.

When I started my training in general surgery over twenty-five years ago, I directly excised the overdeveloped breast tissue through an incision around the edge of the inferior areola. I now use liposuction for this procedure and achieve much smoother outcomes. Occasionally, I might have to directly excise a small amount of tissue, necessitating a slightly larger incision.

## HAIR REMOVAL

Most men seek hair removal for excess hair over their bodies, particularly on the upper back and around the shoulders. Both laser and non-laser light sources are used for this.

A current difficulty with hair removal is that multiple treatments are required for the average patient. Part of the problem is that hair growth involves three phases. If a hunter went out in the winter, he wouldn't be able to shoot a bear because the animal is hibernating in a cave somewhere. Hair also hibernates, and light sources have no effect on sleeping hair follicles.

In the spring, when the follicle wakes up, would be the time for treatment. Trouble is, hair doesn't go through these phases synchronously. So treatments are needed at various times to destroy the hair follicles in different phases. To complicate matters further, the hair follicle or hair shaft sometimes doesn't absorb the light energy.

There are many hair removal systems currently in use. Most rely on damaging color cells in the hair bulb to destroy the hair. Light-colored hair is more difficult to treat and may never be satisfactorily removed. New techniques appear promising, and in my opinion, and some years down the road, complete and permanent hair removal may be a realistic goal.

## IMPLANTS

In men, facial implants are often placed to emphasize the jaw line, elevate cheekbones, or lend prominence to a recessive chin. The only implant I use in men is the chin implant. I don't do cheek or jawline implants or other implants that change the facial structure. Some plastic surgeons, particularly in California, specialize in this extensive profile alteration.

Other implants include pectoralis muscle implants, calf augmentation, and buttock enhancement done with medical-grade elastomer prostheses. Implants have been developed in various sizes and shapes to mimic the pectoralis major muscle and are made out of a soft but solid silicone implant. This is an area where plastic surgery earns its name by actually using plastic.

## LASER RESURFACING

Because men don't use makeup in American society, lasers are used less frequently in males because of the risk of permanent skin color change, a serious concern when doing strong or deep laser treatments. Men's wrinkles tend to run deeper than women's because their skin is thicker, and unfortunately deeper wrinkles demand a stronger laser treatment. Lighter skin around a man's eyes that can't be camouflaged may give him reverse "raccoon-eyes." Skin lightening from laser in general is more common in males, particularly over the forehead area.

## LIPOSUCTION

Liposuction in men generally is done using the ultrasound or power-assisted techniques. Because men's skin is thicker, neck skin in particular will not drape as well as a woman's following liposuction under the chin and neck area. However, for treatment of gynecomastia, ultrasound and power-assisted liposuction have been a wonderful advance. Men also tend to see good results in reducing love handles around the waist and abdomen.

## MALE BROWLIFT

Facial analysis reveals that only a few facial characteristics transform a strong masculine appearance into a more feminine one. One of the most important characteristics is the placement of the brows, including the height and the arch of the brow. The level, flat male eyebrow generally sits lower than the female. A higher, arched eyebrow is distinctly feminine. In males, elevating the eyebrows will feminize the area and can cause a surprised look if the inside of the eyebrow is over-elevated, or a more sinister look if the outside of the eyebrow is overdone.

I rarely perform forehead lifts on men and then only for extreme eyebrow droopiness, called ptosis, or when a patient already has undergone an upper eyelid tuck. Elevation of the eyebrow to a more natural position is generally more successful in these situations, but care must still be taken to avoid the surprised look that can easily occur in the male patient.

A complete and thorough discussion with the patient about the goals of the surgery, precise technical execution, and conservative elevation is needed to end up with a pleasing result that has a natural appearance.

## MALE FACELIFT

Many surgeons modify the incisions when doing a male facelift. Generally, an incision in front of the ear is not brought up into the ear itself because the man's beard could grow into this area and make shaving extremely difficult. Many surgeons overcome this by removing hair follicles. Otherwise, incisions are placed in a crease in front of the ear or along the back edge of the sideburn itself. Behind the ear, the incision is carried quite high, so the ear will conceal most of the scar. The incision then is run straight back into the hair and not along the hairline.

Surgeons instruct male patients to let their hair grow out prior to a facelift, so scars can be camouflaged by hair growth while they fade over the subsequent year. Male skin is thicker and doesn't lend itself to recontouring as easily as female skin, so a crisp neckline following a facelift can't always be achieved.

## PENILE ENLARGEMENT

Penile surgery can be done for either cosmetic or medical reasons. For cosmetic purposes, the ligaments that stabilize the base of the penis can be released with a surgical procedure. This actually lengthens the penis itself. Lipotransfer has been used in the penile area to augment the size of the shaft. Removing an overhanging lower abdomen may not make the penis longer, but it certainly makes it more visible.

Testicular implants can replace a testicle lost because of birth defects, trauma, or surgical removal. They're made of solid silicone and work well. Penile implants are used for impotence most commonly associated with organic disease, including neuropathy that occurs in diabetes, vascular problems such as in atherosclerosis, and neurological problems such as paralysis. Urologists place penile or testicular implants. The device is inflated to cause an erection. Many men opt for surgical implantation of semi-rigid or inflatable devices. Bendable silicone rods may be difficult to conceal because the penis is permanently erect. Inflatable devices work by compressing a pump placed in the scrotum. Complications can include erosion of the device itself, infection, bleeding, and scarring.

## RHINOPLASTY

Most men come to my practice because of breathing problems due to previous nasal fractures, and these concerns certainly should be addressed. Health insurance usually covers surgery to correct breathing problems but not appearance problems. Crooked noses or C-shaped deformities because of previous fractures can be camouflaged in a straightforward manner with modification of the nasal bridge and an onlay of cartilage grafting material.

My goal with a male rhinoplasty patient is to balance the nose overall rather than reducing the underlying nasal structure too much. Refining the nose tip usually involves adding cartilage to give a defining point. Reducing tip cartilage is often fraught with frustration, in my experience, because of scarring and bunching of the skin envelope. Any removal must be conservative. Internal suture techniques to shape the cartilage are very helpful.

## TUMMY TUCK

Abdominoplasty for men emphasizes liposuction and, if necessary, skin excision rather than reinforcing the abdominal muscles, because men don't have their tummy muscles and skin stretched from pregnancy. If possible, I avoid excisional tummy-tuck surgery in men. If I do such surgery, I keep the excision along the pubic hairline and generally avoid detaching the belly button because usually there is not enough excess skin to pull around the umbilicus. If a wide skin excision is necessary, for example in a patient who has had massive weight loss, I tend to modify the procedure by not treating the muscles and excising skin only where necessary.

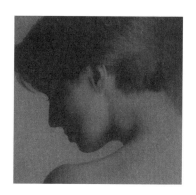

*chapter 10*

# REVISING PLASTIC SURGERY

"Only those who do nothing…make no mistakes."

— Joseph Conrad

*I* tell every patient who comes into my office that they may end up dissatisfied with their procedure and need revisional surgery. Every plastic surgeon occasionally has less than optimal results. This happens in part because plastic surgery is an art, and surgeons are working on a variable canvas, the human body. And sometimes things just don't go as planned even if a procedure was done perfectly, and complications arise. Problems also occur because doctors aren't able to read their patients' minds. Ideas of beauty are intangible, and a patient's concept of larger or smaller or prettier may not be the same as the surgeon's.

I can't emphasize enough the importance of communicating your expectations clearly before any surgery. You also need to listen to your doctor, and realize that your expectations can't always be met. If your doctor tells you that you can only see so much improvement with liposuction instead of a tummy tuck, be realistic about those results.

It is also essential that you read all the material your surgeon gives you before the operation, and that you follow all of the pre- and postsurgical instructions you are given. Ask questions. Understand the pros, cons, and limitations of the procedure you want. If necessary, schedule as many office visits as it takes for you to feel comfortable.

The only way to avoid complications is to not operate. Trouble is inherent in surgery. This is especially true when untrained physicians attempt advanced plastic surgical procedures. The best way to avoid trouble in plastic surgery is for patients to stack the deck in their favor by seeking out plastic surgeons certified by the American Board of Plastic Surgery. An ounce of prevention by doing your homework is worth a pound of surgical revisions later.

Okay, let's say you've experienced a bad result with plastic surgery. The best thing you can do at this point is hang in there. Surgery takes a long time to heal. It might take six months or even a year before you can see the real results of your nose job, facelift or liposuction. Discuss your progress with your doctor at your follow-up visits. Don't immediately start looking for a new surgeon. If you have done your homework and chosen a qualified doctor to begin with, trust that he or she wants you to have the best possible results, and will do what it takes to help you get them.

By sticking with your original surgeon you will probably keep your costs for revisional surgery down. I don't charge my patients for revisions, although a surgical tray or anesthesia fee may be necessary. I do charge full fees for correcting plastic surgery done elsewhere. For instance, 30 percent of the rhinoplasty patients I operate on have had procedures done by other physicians. These patients have to pay another set of surgical fees—but only after I've encouraged them to return to their original surgeons.

Many patients tell me they've lost confidence in their previous practitioners. If this is the case, ask your original surgeon if a close colleague or trusted advisor is available for a second opinion. That way you keep your costs down and keep the lines of communication open, while dealing with the fact that you've lost confidence in the original surgeon.

## KEEP YOUR SURGEON ON YOUR SIDE

Often patients respond to a stressful situation or an untoward result with behavior that alienates the very people who are trying to help them—their original surgeons. Don't get defensive. When patients come in with grocery lists of complaints I try to listen. I feel badly even if I'm not directly to blame for an unexpected healing problem.

My advice to patients is to remain calm. Write down your complaints and stick to the issue. My advice to myself is to listen to patients before I put on my Mr. Fix-It hat. People need to be heard. In picking a surgeon, make sure the person is willing to listen, so that if you have an untoward result you can feel assured that you are working with someone you can communicate with.

If you have lost trust in a doctor who is a solo practitioner, seek the opinion of another surgeon certified by the American Board of Plastic Surgery. You can use the second surgeon as a sounding board for how you feel. After I see a patient who wants a second opinion, I write or call the colleague about the situation. This improves communication and continuity of care.

If the second-opinion surgeon makes you feel more comfortable about your original outcome, you may muster up enough confidence or courage to return to the original surgeon. If not, and you like the second-opinion surgeon, stay put. If you're uncomfortable with both opinions, seek another.

## KNOWING WHEN TO GIVE UP

How do you decide when you've had bad plastic surgery versus an outcome that just hasn't met your expectations? What can be corrected, and when is it time to give up?

### Abdominoplasty, or Tummy Tuck

Touch-up surgery on a fair number of tummy-tuck patients is common. Look for "dog ears" where the end of the incision bulges outward. Additional liposuction and, if necessary, re-excision of excess skin can correct this. However, the trade-off is a longer scar. If you have residual subcutaneous fullness or excess skin following a tummy tuck, this can be easily revised. It's tempting to fix minor wrinkling, irregularities, or malformations of the belly button, but the procedure has the potential to backfire.

Fluid build-up after a tummy tuck is rare. Usually this resolves itself over time with compression and limitation of activity, but a patient may need to have the fluid removed with a needle. On very rare occasions a sac called a pseudobursa that permanently collects fluid may develop. Further surgery is needed to excise the sac lining.

The pubic hairline may be elevated after a tummy tuck. Good patient communication during consultations is important, and your surgeon should make precise preoperative markings so you can agree on where the incisions will be. The pubic hairline moves higher because of tension on the abdominal skin, and this is sometimes a trade-off that needs to be accepted. On the other hand, some patients want this area elevated and sometimes suctioned. Be frank about your expectations and desires.

A complication most often seen with smokers following abdominoplasty is an area of dead abdominal skin. In these cases the skin usually contracts and softens and is less pink a year after surgery. This can be revised with direct excision of the scarred skin in some situations.

Sometimes problems arise because of conditions unrelated to a surgery. I had a 26-year-old patient who had a tummy tuck and breast lift. She was in excellent physical condition and worked out regularly, but due to stressful situations had lost a noticeable amount of weight in the six months since her surgeries. I saw it in her face when I entered the exam room. She complained of excess skin on the sides of her lower abdomen, but this actually was the result of her weight loss. I excised the additional skin, and she accepted the longer surgical scars on each side of her abdomen.

Some problems are simply the result of unrealistic expectations. Sometimes patients will sit forward and complain that they still have rolls in the tummy area. Everyone—even a thin person—has a roll across the lower abdomen when they're sitting. Tummies can only be evaluated in a standing position. If your stomach is completely flat when you're standing, that is the best result you can expect. Patients also can't evaluate their abdomens while moving. They need to be motionless, standing still. If excess tissue is present in this position, then a touch-up could be done.

In some cases, a patient's expectations are simply too high. I once saw a woman who had undergone a tummy tuck in which a new belly button was constructed. She wasn't satisfied with the results and came to me for a second opinion. I could see that her belly button had a little puckering, but I also knew that there was little to be gained from trying to improve on minor imperfections. I told her so and advised her to discuss the situation again with the original doctor.

The woman had additional surgery anyway and came to see me yet again. She now had a scar that was three inches longer on the abdomen, because her original doctor was doing his best to make her happy. She would have been better off not having had more surgery. Maybe her belly button wasn't perfect, but it would have been in her best interest to stop a long time ago. Sometimes a minor problem just isn't worth the price of correcting it.

## Blepharoplasty, or Cosmetic Eyelid Surgery

One of the most dreaded complications of upper eyelid surgery is dry eye syndrome. Removing tissue around the eye opens it up. If your eye is slightly wider, more tears will evaporate. If you are on the border of having dry eyes anyway, this procedure may push them into this extremely uncomfortable situation. I've heard of patients who have to sleep with eyecups and use lubricating drops and ointment during the day.

The best defense against dry eye syndrome is good prevention. A preoperative tear test may be done on patients who complain of dry eyes, and they can be referred to an ophthalmologist for a more extensive tear evaluation. If the patient does indeed have a problem with dry eyes, a surgeon should consider doing either the upper lids or the lower lids with a suspension procedure. All four eyelids should not be done at the same time.

A patient's innate anatomy may cause asymmetry after surgery that can't be corrected. Most other limitations can be fixed. These include fine lines that can be treated and residual fat that can be resected again. The very rare complication of permanent upper lid drooping may need additional surgery to elevate the lid. A pulling down of the lower lid that causes a person to look like a beagle can be corrected with suspension procedures.

### Botox Injection

Occasionally a patient will have severe relaxation of the forehead, called "brow-drop," following a Botox injection. The eyebrows may fall below the edge of the brow bone. There is no antidote to reverse this. The Botox will wear off gradually.

### Breast Augmentation

Breasts that are firmer than the patient wants them to be is the most common problem following breast augmentation. This happens because of the way the patient's body forms scar tissue. Taking vitamin E, doing special exercises, and some new drugs may help. Sometimes, surgery to remove the scar tissue is necessary, but unfortunately there is a 50-50 chance of recurrence.

Another possible problem with breast augmentation is migration of the implant within the pocket—either downward or off to the sides. This can be corrected with plication—a procedure that closes off the overly expanded portion of the implant pocket—or by redefining part of the pocket to reestablish the implant in a more central location.

Almost every patient has a different structure in each of her breasts. Sometimes asymmetries exist preoperatively that can never be surgically corrected. For instance, a patient may have one large breast that has a different shape than a smaller underdeveloped breast. One breast may need to be reduced, but more often the smaller breast is enlarged with an implant. Differences in nipple height may always be present. These types of asymmetries may never be reconciled. The key is to find an experienced surgeon and to lower your expectations. You may never have perfect breasts, but they will look a lot better than they did before the surgery.

A number of patients complain of rippling or wrinkling when implants are placed behind the breast but on top of the muscle The implant itself may wrinkle because of its design. This can be partially corrected by placing the implant under the muscle, affording additional tissue cover. Even in a submuscular pocket, however, many women have wrinkling on the lower outer pole of the breast because muscle usually doesn't cover the area. The rippling may be visible or may only be felt. This is particularly common in thin women who don't have enough subcutaneous tissue to conceal irregularities.

The problem can't be fixed unless you want to gain a lot of weight to give more tissue cover. Most patients can only feel the wrinkles. In my experience, this is not a surgical issue.

Nipple numbness is an uncommon but annoying side effect of surgery. It usually clears up with time but may be permanent and not correctable.

### Breast Lift

Differences from one side to the other in a breast lift often can be corrected. For instance, the outlining of the areola may be slightly larger and can be modified, or fullness in one area compared to another can be alleviated. The breasts will fall again over time, and surgery can be redone.

Many of the problems with initial breast asymmetries discussed in the preceding Breast Augmentation section also apply to this procedure and are not completely correctable.

### Breast Reduction in Women

Problems with irregularities in breast reductions are similar to those with augmentations and lifts. Over-reduction of the breasts can be a problem in a woman with a heavy build, causing her to look like an overweight man rather than a shapely woman. Implants could be placed to re-augment breast size.

Following any breast procedure, the scar could elevate or spread beyond the original incision. These are firm, painful, rock-hard scars that can be treated. An injection with a cortisone preparation every three weeks or so softens and flattens the scar. Silastic inserts can be placed in the bra to help alleviate this problem. Don't accept an elevated red scar; return to your doctor for treatment.

### Browlift

Rarely, a patient may have bad scarring following a browlift. Several of my patients have complained that when the wind blows their hair up, an observer can see visible scars. This may be part and parcel of the procedure, but if the scar is particularly wide your surgeon may be willing to revise it or to revise a bald spot. Follicular unit hair transplants or cosmetic tattooing can also alleviate visible incision scars.

Asymmetry in eyebrow height may occur following the procedure. Your surgeon will have tried to gain symmetry in the level of each eyebrow. This might not have been possible and additional work may need to be done, although sometimes it may be quite difficult or even impossible to achieve near perfection.

### Buttocks Lift

Buttocks may fall again or a scar may widen. Discuss possible revisional surgery with your surgeon. The surgeon will make a clinical judgment about whether additional surgery will yield enough benefits to be worthwhile.

### Cheek Implants

I have seen several patients who are highly dissatisfied with cheek implants. Readjustments are appropriate and, to a point, I would press for revisional surgery if marked asymmetries are visible. A minor deformity may not be correctable and may invite potential problems unless a definitive, straightforward adjustment can be made. My tendency would be to sit tight and not operate.

### Chemical Peels

Skin lightened by a chemical peel can't be corrected. Bleaching creams can alleviate darker areas that may occur following a peel. Of course, additional peeling can always be done, depending on the strength and type of the peel, and may help even out the skin tone.

Many women experience increased blood vessel formation in the neck following peel work, causing a reddened effect. Various experimental laser treatments are being tried, none of which are consistent or reliable. You could request additional work on the neck area to soften the coloration. However, don't be surprised if these efforts yield minimal to no improvement.

### Chin Augmentation

If an implant was used for your chin augmentation procedure, it may become displaced or extrude. This should be corrected. On the other hand, be aware that if you're displeased with your contour and want the implant removed, you may develop a loss of chin support. This may cause droopiness called chin ptosis. This is an extremely difficult and intricate problem to resolve. Few practitioners around the country fully understand the nature of the problem and how to correct it. Think carefully before you decide to have an implant removed. You may create a worse situation for yourself.

Permanent chin numbness is rare and cannot be corrected. Studies on related issues suggest to me that patients may have to wait up to two years before the amount of permanent numbness can be assessed.

### Collagen Injection

The body often absorbs collagen over several months rather than the six to 12 or even 18 months that plastic surgeons and their patients hope for. Occasionally a patient's body will absorb a collagen injection within a matter of weeks. If this occurs, ask your practitioner about an additional injection donated by the manufacturer.

### Dermabrasion

Dermabrasion usually is done to reduce acne scarring or wrinkles and generally can be redone. Some acne scarring is so deep, however, that the surrounding skin can't be smoothed enough without the risk of additional scarring. See a practitioner who has a good deal of experience and conservative judgment in this area. Be prepared to repeat the procedure.

### Facelift

We age in steps. A patient may go through a rapid aging phase and notice excess redundant skin has reaccumulated soon after surgery, perhaps in the first year. Discuss this situation with your practitioner. The surgeon would have to make a clinical judgment about whether improvement could be gained by additional surgery.

A standard facelift won't reduce the skin folds that run between the nose and lips, called the nasal labial folds. This area needs to be addressed with a mid-face lift. Some minor irregularities in the face may never be correctable. On rare occasions, some patients develop prolonged or permanent pain or discomfort in the surgical area that has to be treated with medication.

Elevation of the sideburn area in women can be a problem in facelifts. This can be treated with additional surgery or hair transplantation in unusual situations. A facelift that is too tight isn't correctable, but this would be rare on the first go-round. Again, choose your doctor carefully.

A severe elevated hypertrophic (literally "growing too much") scar or even a keloid scar may sometimes form around some of the incisions, particularly around the back of the ear area following surgery, and your practitioner should treat this aggressively.

### Fat Injection

Fat injections tend to be absorbed. You can always ask for more. However, sometimes the injections are permanent. Puffy areas respond to massage.

### Gynecomastia Treatment

Residual areas of fullness or asymmetries following male breast reduction can be touched up with additional liposuction or, when necessary, direct excision. Within limits—and assuming a marked difference doesn't exist from one side of the chest to the other—most men can expect a pretty good symmetrical result. Minor differences from one side to the other cannot be improved with surgery, and actually are far more common in the human body than total symmetry. Be sure your expectations are realistic and don't let yourself obsess about absolute perfection.

### Hair Transplantation

The main concern with hair transplantation is that you might need additional hair to fill out the area where the transplants were placed. Discuss this with your surgeon. Ask about any recent medical or surgical developments.

### Laser Skin Resurfacing

Touch-up surgery on facial areas with extremely deep wrinkles is common following laser skin resurfacing. As with chemical peels, darker areas can be treated with bleaching creams. An area of skin that has been bleached by the laser can't be improved, and makeup or cosmetic tattooing would be necessary.

A particularly vexing problem following laser surgery is a color step-off—a change in color where the visual border of the jawline meets the neck skin, for example. There is no solution.

### Laser Treatment of Leg Veins

Dark areas on the leg can be caused by laser treatments. They can be treated with bleaching cream but may never be completely resolved. Severe discoloration sometimes occurs, and no reliable treatment is available. This potential risk should be fully discussed and accepted by the patient prior to the procedure. Smokers can experience skin loss, in which the skin dies. This produces even more discoloration. Don't smoke! Secondary treatments for leg veins are commonplace.

### Lip Augmentation

Asymmetrical areas following lip augmentation may occur and, unless they were present preoperatively, could be correctable. Preoperative asymmetries are difficult to fully correct, and you may need to lower your expectations. An asymmetry that appears to have been caused by the surgery can be verified by carefully reviewing pre-operative and postoperative photographs. This most likely is correctable. Ask your surgeon's opinion. Additional material can always be inserted in the lip area.

### Liposuction

Leftover areas of fullness are the most common problem following liposuction; in fact the cost of touch-up surgery sometimes may be folded into the initial procedure by your surgeon because it is so often needed. Feel free to request a touch-up or enhancement. Even if your surgeon's fee includes touch-ups, however, be aware that you will still have to pay any surgical center charges.

Sometimes the reverse happens, and an area of indentation or a localized depression is what is actually making an area look too full. Perhaps adding fat to the surrounding area will smooth out the contour. This, of course, is an artistic, clinical judgment that must be made for each patient.

Ligaments that hold up the buttocks and back may relax following liposuction, causing a banana-shaped deformity or double buttock crease fold. This is a real problem and isn't easily correctable. Be patient with your practitioner. If the surgeon is willing to operate again on this area, there may still be only some correction possible. This problem is most likely to occur if you have a lot of fat removed from these areas.

**Liposuction is not a weight-loss procedure.** If you're dissatisfied overall with your surgical result, you may want to inquire about the volume removed. You may want a second opinion, but keep in mind the procedure is designed to alleviate localized contour fullness in areas with excellent overlying skin tone. Liposuction is not a substitute for diet and exercise but a complement to it. I try to sculpt the abdomen and even try to give the patient the appearance of a "six pack" or an indentation down the midline if that's what she wants, but it doesn't always work out.

Bagginess and the settling of inelastic skin is a potential problem and isn't always predictable on preoperative examination. If liposuction on your neck leaves turkey skin behind, you may need a full facelift. Prolonged bruising is another problem that can occur, especially on the outside of the thighs. This doesn't seem to relate directly to surgical technique. Once bruising is there, it just takes time to go away.

## Otoplasty, or Cosmetic Ear Surgery

Correct diagnosis, careful planning, and precise surgical execution can avoid many problems that follow otoplasty. Prevention is much easier than revision. If a patient is dissatisfied despite what a surgeon thinks is a good outcome, the problem can often be traced to expectations that weren't communicated clearly during preoperative consultations.

Otoplasty generally is done to set back a cup ear deformity. Ideally, from a front view, both ears should be clearly visible and their rims should be slightly outside the inner ear fold. During the procedure, a surgeon needs to evaluate how far out from the head the ear is and how it looks, keeping in mind the need for symmetry with the opposite side. I often use a ruler to measure the top, middle, and bottom of one ear for comparison to the other. A gentle curve should be achieved.

Over-correction, or a "pinned-back" appearance, is difficult, if not impossible, to correct. It's essential to tell—or show—your surgeon how far back you want your ears before surgery. I give my patients mirrors before they enter the operating room and gradually push back each ear to the point where they are satisfied. I then measure this, make a note of it, and replicate it during the procedure.

Unfortunately, cup ear deformity may reoccur. A touch-up procedure might bring the ear back toward the head to reestablish symmetry. A small symmetrical difference between sides is probably not worth the effort of surgery and may not be correctable anyway. Discuss the situation with your practitioner, but keep an open mind and realize the limitations when you start talking about a small difference from one side to the other.

A telephone deformity occurs when the central portion of the ear is farther toward the head than the upper and lower portions of the ear. Occasionally removal of a small crescent of skin or fat from the backside of the earlobe will set it into better contour. Protruding earlobes and upper ears that stick out from the head are amenable to additional surgery.

A severe elevated keloid scar may sometimes form around the ear area following surgery, and your practitioner should treat this aggressively. An irregularity from the sutures isn't a significant problem that needs to be treated. Draining sutures, however, should be pursued aggressively and removed if the patient suffers continued irritation.

### Rhinoplasty, or Nose Reshaping

Fifteen percent of rhinoplasty surgeries need to be revised. Pick your doctor very, very, very carefully. I revise my own patients, usually at no charge. If I do a secondary procedure on a patient whose original surgery was done elsewhere, I have to charge full fees. In some cases I even charge more because the situation is more complicated than doing it the first time.

Develop a relationship with a doctor you feel is frank and honest. If something is obviously wrong, and your practitioner passes it off, seek a second opinion from an experienced nasal surgeon. If you have a minimal or minor deformity, it might be best to accept this.

Occasionally a hole deep inside the septal area develops following rhinoplasty. This is referred to as a septal perforation and may show itself through a whistling sound when a patient breathes during sleep or by continued crusting and drainage from inside the nose. Septal perforation is very rare and very difficult to correct. If it isn't causing problems, no surgery will be done. If it is, discuss this with your surgeon. You may need to be referred to a highly skilled specialist for correction.

Rarely, patients develop breathing problems following cosmetic rhinoplasty. Additional grafting may be necessary to the internal or external nasal valves to promote breathing. You may have to accept the fact that the mid-portion of your nose may be slightly wider following a correction involving internal valves. There also may be some internal blockage, and this should be thoroughly evaluated.

Occasionally patients complain of postnasal drip they didn't have prior to cosmetic rhinoplasty. Sometimes this can be fixed with surgery, so I do a thorough exam to see if a problem with irregularity, redundant mucosa, scarring, or excess tissue might be the culprit. If no significant problems are found, the patient may have to adjust and accept the situation. Sometimes nasal sprays help.

Adding grafting material when redoing nasal surgery is very, very common. If you have had nose surgery and still feel your nose is too big, don't be surprised if your surgeon wants to add grafts to your nose when all you want to do is subtract something. Most of the time, the key to revisional nasal surgery is to add something—with the net result being better balance and proportion.

If your surgeon explains you have extremely thick skin and additional work will not help you, believe it. Thick, scarred skin severely limits a surgeon in obtaining refinement in nasal surgery. That doesn't mean a surgeon won't try, but it will be difficult, if not impossible, to achieve all of the hoped-for results.

### Scars

It's difficult to hit a home run on scar revision surgery. Wide scars or scars that are elevated, firm, pink, and tender can—and should—be treated. Persist with your desire to improve these things, and you will be rewarded. However, if a practitioner doesn't feel a scar can be improved beyond a certain point, accept the opinion. For example, a wide scar located over a joint is likely to recur because of continued motion and tension. Once skin is cut, a scar is permanent. Sometimes it can be made less noticeable, but it can never be made invisible. Silicone gel sheeting can be helpful.

### Thigh Lift

Problems specific to thigh lifts include scar migration, which is difficult to correct. Discuss with your surgeon whether it's possible to move the inferior skin upward into the groin crease to hide the scar better. Labial separation in a woman, particularly when a patient bends or stoops, can be a chronic problem.

Early recurrence of baggy skin may occur following a thigh lift. Evaluate yourself in a standing position—not lying on your side or in a posture that induces the problem. Additional skin can be excised but be cautious because extreme tension in this area can cause labial separation. You may have to accept some limitations on the corrections possible in this area.

### Upper Arm Lift

This procedure basically is designed to remove excess skin and subcutaneous tissue from the posterior, or back side, of the upper arm. Hypertrophic scarring—where a scar is elevated, pink, firm, and tender—is a potential problem. Silicone sheeting and, possibly, cortisone injections can ease this. Localized areas of contour fullness can be liposuctioned. It's unusual to re-excise lax skin in this area, but I have done so on occasion. Injecting fat into the area may soften a depression.

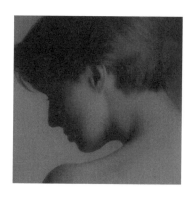

*chapter 11*

# TAKING CARE OF

# YOUR SKIN

"Surgery isn't for everybody.
Whether you're contemplating or have had facial surgery,
an adequate skin care program is necessary
to look younger. Every face is an aging face."

– Anonymous

$\mathcal{T}$he single most important action you can take to maintain a youthful appearance is to avoid the sun. The skin absorbs the sun's energy. Patients with lighter skin are at the most risk for skin malignancies and wrinkles.

Ultraviolet-A (UVA) rays penetrate the skin and are the chief cause of wrinkling. They create that leathery look, sunspots, and overall photo-aging changes. Recently, studies have shown that UVA rays help induce the three most common skin cancers. Short-wavelength solar rays—ultraviolet-B or UVB—are most potent in causing sunburn and are considered the main cause of all types of skin cancer. Sunscreens chemically absorb or block UV rays.

## SUNSCREENS AND SUNBLOCKS

Forget what you've learned about sunscreens. It's all outdated. Previous sunscreens—even though they advertised that they blocked UVA and UVB rays—didn't block the full spectrum of these rays. Although this isn't proven, the increased incidence of malignancies has led dermatologists to speculate that sunscreens actually didn't block the rays of the sun's spectrum that cause melanomas. Because people wore sunscreens, they assumed that they could remain outdoors for longer periods of time, but they were actually exposing themselves to more of the rays that cause potentially fatal skin malignancies.

Sun protection factor, or SPF, measures the time a product protects against skin reddening from UVB rays—compared to how long skin takes to redden without protection. If it takes 20 minutes without protection, using an SPF 15 sunscreen allows 15 times the exposure. You should always use a sunscreen with SPF 15 or higher. Be sure whatever you use blocks all types of rays. Sunscreens need to be applied about 20 minutes before sun exposure, so they can sink into skin layers and bond with surrounding tissue.

A sunblock is stronger than a sunscreen. It physically deflects ultraviolet rays and is completely effective immediately upon application. To block a substantial portion of the full spectrum of UVA and UVB, the best bet is to use a sunscreen that contains zinc oxide or titanium dioxide. Zinc oxide is that white pasty stuff you see on lifeguards' noses. Manufacturers now have developed a means to suspend this in a solution that is clear when applied to skin.

If you sweat heavily, gels stay on much better than creams. Find a gel that contains avobenzone or Parsol, ingredients that block the full spectrum of UVA and lots of UVB rays. Water-resistant sunscreens are great, but because they contain additional ingredients they may sting your eyes.

We all know the sun's rays are strongest at midday, and sun exposure should be avoided between 10 a.m. and 4 p.m. Wear protective clothing and sunglasses and stay in the shade during these hours. Remember, the sun's rays reflect from asphalt, sidewalks, beach sand, and lake water. That's why it's easy to get sunburned even if you're wearing a broad-brimmed hat and sitting under a beach umbrella. Always use sunscreen. It's a good idea to reapply sunscreen every two hours, and, of course, right after swimming.

## INDOOR TANNING

The electric beach still is a form of radiation. Indoor tanning with or without burning causes photo-aging and an increased incidence of skin cancers. Multiple studies have concluded that tanning, not just burning, can cause skin damage and skin cancers. The Federal Trade Commission requires product labels with warnings about tanning.

## SMOKING AND SKIN

If you are a smoker, the second best thing you can do to protect your skin from premature aging, after avoiding sun exposure, is to quit smoking. Smoking directly affects the skin's ability to regenerate and rejuvenate itself. It promotes loss of elasticity, resulting in multiple, deep wrinkles.

A study by dermatologists published in the British medical journal *Lancet* shows smoking activates genes responsible for an enzyme that breaks down collagen in the skin. Collagen is the main structural protein of the skin and keeps it elasticized. When it starts to disintegrate, skin begins to sag and wrinkle.

Other studies have described "smoker's face," in which the breakdown of the skin's elastic fibers gives rise to yellow, irregularly thickened skin. Cigarette smoke damages collagen and elastin in lung tissue and may cause changes in smokers' skin by similar mechanisms. Clinical changes in smokers' skin, including a gray tint and prominent wrinkling, may be due to these changes, according to one study.

The vascular structure of the skin may also play a role. Because smoking constricts the skin's vascular structure, decreased blood flow may induce local skin irritation and carry more toxic substances to these tissues. The skin is weakened, and it wrinkles, the theory goes.

Some researchers think the effects of smoking and sun damage may be synergistic. In any case, alone or together, both are bad for your skin. You should avoid them all the time, and be especially aware of the increased risks from smoking and the sun if you are having cosmetic surgery.

## A SKIN CARE PROGRAM

Many excellent skin care programs are available. Generally, a skin care program involves a cleanser followed by a conditioning solution that opens pores. If necessary, acne medication is applied at this point. A vitamin C-based cell restorer also can be applied. Vitamin E also helps restore the skin, as well as directly protecting skin from the harmful effects of solar radiation. (Recent studies have discovered using both vitamin C and E together has a synergistic effect that can actually undo harmful effects, thus decreasing your chances of developing skin cancer. The actual radiation fractures to skin DNA can be repaired to some degree. This is exciting news.)

Next, a rejuvenator is applied. As people age, skin cells are manufactured only half as fast as when a person is younger. Everything you've heard about Retin-A, alpha hydroxy acids, and Renova is true. These and other new compounds like copper peptides speed up cell turnover, and that can make your skin look younger. Unfortunately they also tend to dry the skin. Some cause redness, burning, peeling, and irritation. In a skin care regimen, the rejuvenating agents can be applied, then a sunscreen. One way to remember that the sunscreen goes on last is to recall that the outer layer is closest to the sun.

## Tips for Maintaining Youthful, Healthy Skin

- Wear protective clothing or use a sunscreen or sunblock whenever you will be exposed to the sun.

- Stay out of tanning booths.

- Do not smoke.

- Follow a regular skin care program.

- Maintain a healthy diet including whole grains breads, fruits and vegetables.

- Exercise regularly.

Proper diet and exercise also help people remain more youthful—not just physiologically but cosmetically. It isn't clear why our skin ages exactly, but doctors and scientists speculate that free radicals are involved. Specific vitamins are free radical scavengers. Whole grain breads, fruits, and vegetables contain these valuable vitamins. The Sears' *Zone* diet discussed in the appendix also markets skin care products that keep your skin "in *The Zone.*" Exercise increases circulation to the skin and gives it a healthy, rosy glow and a more youthful appearance.

There are a multitude of treatments to enhance the skin, my favorites being Intense Pulsed Light (IPL) to blend sun-damaged color changes to the skin, and citric acid peels or kojic acid for mild ongoing skin rejuvenation. Many patients complain to me about the high cost and low yield of microdermabrasion. Don't expect anything more than softer skin or you will definitely be disappointed.

Even if you don't want to take the plunge with cosmetic surgery, you can do a lot to take care of your skin by avoiding the sun and combining healthy living habits with a state-of-the-art skin care program.

## SKIN CANCERS

There are three general types of skin cancer. The first is a *basal cell carcinoma*. This cancer rarely spreads. This is a bad-news/good-news situation. Patients do have cancer, but it's curable. "If you have to have cancer, this is the one to get," I tell patients.

A basal cell carcinoma usually has raised, pearly white edges and a depressed center. It may bleed and then heal, bleed and re-heal. It is slow-growing but is best removed when small so less scarring occurs.

A *squamous cell carcinoma* is a step up the severity ladder. This form of cancer can spread to the lymph nodes in the head and neck area. Squamous cell carcinoma appears more like an ulcer or open sore. It's quite common on the ears or the lower lip. Basal cell cancer is more common on the upper lip. No one knows why.

Finally, there is *malignant melanoma*. Melanomas are increasing, and it doesn't appear to be because of better screening methods or higher awareness. There is just a higher incidence of melanoma. Sydney, Australia, has the highest melanoma rate per person in the world. It also has the most hours of sunlight of any city in the world.

On the other hand, more melanomas are being discovered early, before they develop deep roots and spread around the body. This has caused the mortality rate to drop rapidly. There are now clinics that specialize in melanomas.

Watch any skin lesions or growths for any type of change. A suspicious attitude is a good thing when it comes to cancer. Look for the three Bs—bigger, blacker, or bleeding—and if you notice any one of them, have a physician check it out. Many physicians have biopsies performed on any growth they suspect is cancerous.

Skin cancer rarely strikes people younger than 18 years old. Cases have been reported, but it's extremely rare. Children basically don't get skin cancer unless they have large hairy moles present at birth. Smaller moles that are present at birth do have a very slight chance of becoming cancerous later in life. These should be removed, but there's no rush. I waited until my daughter was 12 years old and could hold still, so her suspicious birth mole could be removed with novocaine rather than general anesthesia.

## VENUS FREEZE®

Venus Freeze® is the first FDA-cleared aesthetic technology, and is a technology that combines Multi-Polar Radio Frequency and Pulsed Magnetic Fields to deliver effective treatments that are painless and require no downtime. Radiofrequency and Magnetic Pulses have been used in medicine for many years and are proven, safe and effective technologies.

Venus Freeze® is used to treat wrinkles, tighten skin and reduce cellulite. The face, neck, and entire body can be treated with Venus Freeze®. The results will be a tightening of the skin, softening of wrinkles, plumper, fuller and overall a more youthful appearance.

The number of treatments required will vary from patient to patient, but typically 5 treatments for the face and neck and 8 treatments for the body.

## HYDRAFACIAL®

HydraFacial® provides cleansing, exfoliation, extractions, and hydration, including Vortex-Fusion® of antioxidants, peptides, and hyaluronic acid. The HydraFacial® is a non-invasive, non-surgical procedure that delivers instant results with no discomfort or downtime. You can see improvement in sun damage, dry skin, hyperpigmentation, fine lines, wrinkles, skin clarity, resilience and firmness. HydraFacial® also works well for oily and acne-prone skin, congested skin and enlarged pores. Homecare products can be used to optimize your results.

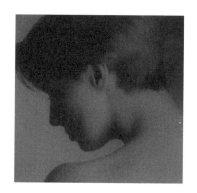

*chapter 12*

# THE REST OF THE HEALTH AND BEAUTY PICTURE: DIET, EXERCISE AND SKIN CARE

"What most of us struggle with isn't what to do
but the motivation to do anything at all."

– Dr. Joe

$\mathcal{A}$s a plastic surgeon I can do artistic things to the outside of your body to refine your beauty, help regress aging, and define your shape. After I complete my work, what happens on the inside of your body dictates long-term success on the outside. You are in charge of that inside success. Diet, exercise, and skin care are the keys.

Diet, exercise, and skin care are endlessly detailed in magazines, books, airwaves, fine fashion stores, and support groups across the world. Every woman, it seems, has a favorite regimen to trim pounds, stay in shape, and care for her complexion. Many women have tried hundreds of programs to achieve their goals. Many people are deeply frustrated with the outcomes.

In this chapter I remind you of some genuinely healthy self-care basics. Whatever your personal regimen, you can keep the basics in mind. I then share my personal diet, exercise, and skin care program.

## DIET

You are what you eat. You also are when you eat, how you eat, how often you eat, what balance of foods you eat, what vitamins you take, how much fat you eat, and your own chemistry and genetics.

For years the standard of ideal weight was reported on the government weight chart, which indicated a range of weight supposedly appropriate to a particular height. It wasn't a very realistic chart because it didn't take into consideration a number of factors, including fitness (muscle weighs a little more than fat), age, bone density, or body type.

Over the past ten years the medical community has replaced the old weight charts with a far more reliable tool: *body mass index.* The BMI measures the ratio of weight to size and takes into account those factors left out of the old charts. It is easy to calculate your BMI using this formula:

$$\text{Body Mass Index (BMI)} = \frac{\text{Weight in pounds}}{(\text{Height in inches}) \times (\text{Height in inches})} \times 703$$

For the average adult a BMI under 18.5 is too thin. The normal range is 19–25. Overweight is 26–30, and anything over 30 is obese. You'll find BMI calculators on the internet if you prefer not to do the math.

The important thing is to monitor your BMI rather than your weight. Your BMI gives you a more accurate picture of your weight as an expression of fitness and self-care.

Food is simultaneously an incredibly complex subject and a very simple one. People have extremely intricate relationships with food. It affects our lives in emotional, financial, physical, social, psychological, and chemical ways. Most people devote a great deal of time and attention to shopping, preparation, serving, eating, and cleaning up after meals. The industries that create kitchen implements, recipe books, and cooking accessories are huge. Fortunes have been made by authors of diet books. We are a people obsessed with food.

Food can also be an "enemy" to many people who battle to lose weight or keep weight stable. Sadly, we are an increasingly obese nation. Too many people lose their battles with food.

Said simply, our bodies require a certain amount of fuel to keep going. Fuel comes in the forms of carbohydrates, proteins, and fats. Our digestive systems break down most food into glucose—the body's fuel. Glucose is simple sugar. If there's too much glucose, the body stores the extra as short-term fuel in both the liver and the muscles. Long-term storage converts glucose into fat. The simple truth is too much fuel in any form – carbohydrates, proteins, or fats—gets stored in the

**The Pasta Diet
(It really works!)**

---

- You walk pasta the bakery...

- You walk pasta the candy store...

- You walk pasta the ice cream shop...

- You walk pasta the table and fridge.

You will lose weight!

–Anonymous

body; it ultimately gets stored in fat cells. If you want to reduce what's in storage, you need to reduce the fuel intake (eat less) and/or increase the fuel used (exercise more).

Here's where all the diet plans in the world begin: reducing the intake. Millions of people used to meticulously keep track of every calorie they consumed, aiming for the magic daily total which would melt those fat cells.

Nutritional science has evolved a long way in the past ten years. Researchers now look not only at what we eat, but also at how and when our bodies process what we eat. This would be the Holy Grail for the perfect combination of optimal health and weight management. Most foods now have labels which reveal the calories and nutritional elements of the food in the package. Whatever diet plan you follow, learn to read the labels and pay attention to the contents of what you eat.

Personally, I follow the nutritional plan of Dr. Barry Sears. He calls it *The Zone Diet* (also see Chapter 13). Dr. Sears teaches a system for eating which incorporates the hormonal and enzyme tides of our bodies. I found *The Zone Diet* after experimenting with many other systems. I find it easy to follow and easy to incorporate into my lifestyle—very important qualities of a good nutritional plan. *The Zone Diet* is a healthy approach to managing weight and nutrition which has been very successful for thousands of people in the nation, including me, my wife, and many of our friends.

### Practicality

*The Zone Diet* is easy to incorporate into your real world. While some more extreme diets may take weight off quite quickly, they don't help you learn to approach eating differently. The weight seems to come back as rapidly as it left when you return to a "regular" life. *Practicality*, therefore, is an important quality of a good diet system.

### Balance

Another important quality in a good diet is *balance*. We are physically engineered to be omnivores, to eat broadly from proteins, carbohydrates, and fats. Our bodies expect a range of foods to supply various nutrients. When your diet restricts variety or leans too heavily on one food group, your body becomes chemically unbalanced.

Our bodies are resilient and can manage a short period of depravation, but eating a highly unbalanced diet for a long period of time can have serious or even dire consequences. From a practical point of view, it's also hard to maintain such a diet because boredom sets in and overwhelms focus.

In addition to a balanced intake of foods, we also need to be certain our diets provide a balance of vitamins and minerals. There is a special group of vitamins which are particularly important. These nutrients have the ability to attach to non-nutritional elements in our bodies and prevent them from doing damage. These vitamins are called *antioxidants* since they attach to oxidized byproducts (free radicals) which can cause aging and disease in the body.

The antioxidant vitamins are A, C, and E. Think ACE. Vitamin A appears in green, leafy veggies. Vitamin C is in citrus fruits especially, but also in other fruits and fresh veggies. Vitamin E comes from grains. These powerful vitamins also slow down aging.

Fortunately, we can obtain vitamins and minerals from supplements as well as from food, but remember a vitamin tablet doesn't substitute for a great fruit salad, natural protein, or healthy grain product. Vitamins are absorbed best when your digestive system is working on food, so take your vitamins with meals.

There are many other vitamins and minerals which are important for a healthy balance in our diets. You can find information about all of them through research in books or the Internet, or by consulting a nutritionist.

### Endurability

*Endurability* is a third quality of a good eating plan. When you consider a diet, ask yourself if you can follow the plan for more than a few days. Is there enough variety? Is there enough flexibility? Can you live with it? If you can't, you won't stick with it.

### Healthiness

*Healthiness* is the fourth quality of a potent diet. I remember a lot of goofy diets I've heard or read about: the egg and grapefruit diet, the cabbage soup diet, the persimmon diet, the all-yogurt diet and thousands more. What they all had in common was a severe restriction of choice and quantity. Our bodies can endure depravation for a short time, and most of these radical diets were intended for short-term use.

What is worrisome, however, is denying basic nutrition. Even for short periods, poor diet and poor nutrition upsets the chemical balance of our bodies and amounts to taking an unnecessary risk. We want our bodies to absorb those chemicals—in the proper amounts—which make our heart, lungs, nervous system, liver, kidneys, and blood do their jobs smoothly and efficiently.

Over our lives, we're going to make some really bad dietary decisions. Who doesn't want a slice of cheesecake or a warm brownie every once in a while? The object is to make poor choices infrequently and to compensate for them by choosing the best nutrition as often as we can.

Just a brief comment about *anorexia* and *bulimia* - these are eating disorders. These are extremes of behavior regarding the restriction or elimination of food. We currently have an epidemic of eating disorders concurrent with the epidemic of obesity in our nation.

Neither anorexia nor bulimia is a "diet." They are, instead, behavioral expressions of mental disorders and are best addressed by mental health practitioners along with nutritional management. The people who deprive themselves of healthy nutrition in such extreme ways are engaged in a very deadly battle. Their lives are, quite literally, at stake. If you are attempting to starve your body to an unreasonable size and shape, I really encourage you to seek help and get yourself back in healthy control.

The reward for healthy eating is health, and you can't beat that! Your objective should be to find a nutritional regimen you can comfortably live with while your body arrives at its ideal shape and size. Once you have achieved this, you can further improve the package with exercise.

## EXERCISE

Cardio, fat burning, toning, shaping, aerobics, dance, swimming, walking, marathons, jogging, horseback riding, skating, skiing, weight lifting, and power shopping: All of these activities—any activity—will benefit flexibility, strength, endurance, toning, muscle control, and cardio-pulmonary health. As a side benefit, exercise causes our bodies to achieve an optimal state of weight and size, and we even live longer.

Just as there is an ocean of info about weight loss, there is a sea of information about exercise. Your choices are nearly infinite to get your muscles moving. What most of us struggle with isn't *what* to do, but the motivation to do anything at all.

Exercise is hard work—it's the work that benefits our bodies. Just as we're engineered to eat diverse foods, our bodies are engineered to perform physical labor. Exercise makes our hearts pump, our lungs expand, and our muscles work. It also makes our bones stronger because stronger bones are needed to anchor stronger muscles. Strong bones are critical for women because women have a higher risk of osteoporosis, a sharp decrease in bone density accompanying aging. Osteoporosis is genetically linked, but can be controlled with a diet rich in calcium and vitamin D and with weight-bearing exercise to strengthen the muscles and bones.

As in all things, balance is very important in exercise. If you only lift weights, for example, you may have strength and toning, but your cardio-pulmonary health isn't optimal. If you only jog, your cardio-pulmonary status might be great and you'll have endurance but your strength and overall toning might be lacking. An ideal exercise program mixes strength, cardio-pulmonary, toning, and fat-burning elements.

Each person's body will require different exercises to achieve this balance. Some of this has to do with genetics since our body types dictate what we need. It also has to do with experience. If we have been very fit in childhood, then we will need a different program to maintain fitness than someone who has not been fit before.

There is good news. With the infinite possibilities for getting yourself moving, something has to appeal to you. More good news: Our bodies respond quickly to exercise. Even if you've been a total couch potato and can barely get onto a treadmill, you can begin walking at a pace which gets your pulse up and your blood flowing. The next time it's not so hard to get onto the treadmill. You can go a bit faster until eventually you're bounding onto the treadmill and jogging or running. All this is at your own pace.

Exercise science and physiology continue to provide us with programs and products to help us get fit without injury. You're more likely to continue working out if you're not injured or in pain.

If you belong to a health club, you'll find well-trained experts. They are available to help you set up a program tailored to improve your fitness without injury or pain. It's a great idea to spend a bit of money to work with a trainer if you're just beginning a program of exercise. He or she will help you learn how to pace yourself, how to use each of the machines which round out your workout, and best of all will provide words of encouragement to help you keep going.

I am proud to be exercise-committed. I have run marathons in Boston, New York, Chicago, and Minneapolis, and I have done some non-competitive running at high altitudes. I am currently training year-round for extreme cross-country skiing. I also bike and swim.

I began my commitment to exercise after back surgery when I was a teenager. What started as physical therapy became and continues to be a part of my life. Even during the rigors of medical school and my residency, I always found time to exercise, as I continue to do today.

What works for me may not be right for you. You have to discover your own program, which is best judged by your level of fitness, how you feel during and after exercise, and your ability to commit to it. It doesn't really matter what you do as long as you do something, do it regularly, and do it for life!

## MY PERSONAL HEATH RITUALS: DIET AND EXERCISE

I start every day with a *Zone* diet "big brain" shake. Sure, go ahead and have a cup of coffee, too. My shake balances protein, carbs, and fat consistent with *The Zone Diet*. I pour blueberries (lots), raspberries, blackberries, strawberries, grapes (dark purple, red, green), and cranberry juice into the blender. If I have apples, cantaloupe, honeydew, or pineapple, I will add these extras too. Next I add a small carrot and small amounts of baby spinach, romaine lettuce, celery, broccoli, and cauliflower. The more colorful the palette of fruits and vegetables, the more antioxidants are available.

Antioxidants bind the nasty free radicals in your system. As a result they retard aging and inhibit precancerous cells. Your daily requirement for fruit and vegetables is instantly filled, and you have a great start on your total daily fiber requirement of 25 grams.

Researchers have developed a rating scale that measures the antioxidant potency of foods and supplements. The scale measures Oxygen Radical Absorbance Capacity (ORAC). The colorful plant group of fruits and vegetables has up to 20 times the antioxidant power of other foods and vitamins. Aromatic essential oils are also powerful antioxidants, and many of them can act as food supplements. High ORAC prevents aging. Animals fed high-ORAC foods had lower biological ages. Some physicians believe antioxidant power correlates with cancer prevention. I certainly do.

### Since You Must Eat, Make Food a Drug

I recommend a minimum of 3,000 ORAC units per day. Since a cup of blueberries contains almost 5,000 ORAC units, you should have no problem using these foods to stay younger and healthier. The ORAC values of the top antioxidant foods are available on-line from the U.S. Department of Agriculture. You will be happy to know dark chocolate (which actually raises your endorphins) and unprocessed cocoa powder are among the foods with the highest ORAC. All the ingredients of my breakfast shake are ORAC superfoods. If you have to eat anyway, you might as well make food a drug.

Finally I add a calculated amount (mine is 28 grams) of protein powder. Dr. Sears outlines this easy protein calculation for you. I prefer soy protein because it reduces cardiovascular disease.

For my "good" fat (monounsaturated fat) requirement, I toss in an ounce of almonds and a teaspoon of olive oil. I blend this tasty breakfast and enjoy the shake's rich fruity flavor. I also take vitamin and mineral supplements, including selenium, lycopene and a tablespoon of medical-grade fish oil for my long-chain omega-3 fatty acids to prevent inflammation. Flax seed oil also provides omega fatty acids.

I am a big label-reader, watching out for destructive trans-fatty acids. If you read the words "partially hydrogenated" with any ingredient on the label, then trans-fatty acids are present. If there are less than 0.5 grams of trans-fatty acids in the food, then the label, by law, can claim there is no trans-fat present. Don't be fooled into eating small amounts of trans-fatty acids when you were led to believe you are eating healthy.

*Hesperidin*, a natural phytonutrient extract from fruit, can dramatically increase your good cholesterol (HDL—high-density lipoprotein). When all is said and done, if you use these healthy practices (including regular exercise), and still have trouble with your cholesterol levels (serum lipids), ask your family doctor if you might benefit from a statin medication. Statins are a class of drugs that reduces serum cholesterol levels.

Scientific research predicts the two things most likely to shorten my life span are prostate cancer and cardiovascular disease. Eskimo men don't develop prostate cancer. Their high consumption of fish oil has been linked to preventing prostate cancer. I make sure to take a tablespoon of pharmaceutical-grade fish oil every day. If your triglycerides are high, fish oil will level them out dramatically. My preventive cardiologist also recommends I take extra daily Folate (1200 mcg. total), B6 (50 mg.) and B12 (500 mcg.) to prevent heart attacks.

I keep up on my regular aerobic exercise. Lifting weights helps tone my muscles to build strength for posture and balance. Studies demonstrate the additional benefits from weight lifting include: stronger bones (less osteoporosis), less heart disease, and better vision as you grow older.

People break a hip more from the impact of the fall than directly from weak bones secondary to osteoporosis. So a lack of balance is the overriding concern. Do you realize your balance can actually be trained? Try standing with your toes of one foot right behind the heel of your other foot. Hold your arms 90 degrees straight out from the sides of your body. Next, close your eyes, and see how long you can maintain this position. Practice this exercise to lengthen how long you can stay in this position. Try to get to the point where you can stand like this indefinitely. You could also invest in a balance board and practice balance while reading.

I try to keep my mind young. Alzheimer's disease is thought by some medical researchers to be the result of an inflammatory process. Fish oil is a natural anti-inflammatory. Therefore fish oil would help to inhibit this inflammation and has no side effects.

You can actually grow new neuronal connections in your brain for your entire life, regardless of age. Working cross-word puzzles is the most widely advertised method of keeping your mind sharp. Combining a motor skill along with a mental challenge, like playing a musical instrument, ballroom dancing, or cross-country skiing, is even more effective. Cross-country skiing in the winter or roller skiing in the summer demands crisp technique and sharp concentration. I form new coordination pathways by practicing. It also requires a tremendous amount of balance. Some studies demonstrate it is the most demanding aerobic exercise. So by a single activity, I benefit from all three challenges: a mental challenge, balance training, and aerobic exercise.

Overall the single best thing you can do for yourself is to not smoke. Based on recent findings the second best thing you can do to live longer and healthier is to maintain your blood pressure below 115/75. Avoiding salt and exercising regularly will help you maintain a healthy blood pressure. I practice biofeedback, prayer, meditation and positive

## My Personal Big Picture Outline

- Eat fruits and vegetables each day
- Eat plenty of fiber
- Add soy protein to your diet
- Drink 8 ounces of water each hour during the day
- Drink spring water or filtered water whenever possible
- Take vitamins, minerals, and selenium
- Avoid trans-fats
- Take Hesperidin capsules daily
- Take fish oil supplements daily
- Do aerobic exercise
- Do weight lifting
- Do balance exercises (e.g., balance on one foot waiting in line to buy groceries)
- Do mind-stretching exercises
- Don't smoke
- Keep your blood pressure under 115/75
- Do biofeedback, prayer, or meditation for at least 20 minutes daily
- Do something kind for someone else every day

visualization each day for twenty minutes to keep my blood pressure down, dialogue and listen to God, and take an inventory of my life. Celery seed capsules can control more persistent blood-pressure issues.

I also want to stress the importance of drinking plenty of water. Recent articles claim that drinking too much water can be dangerous. In my own life, I find two telling experiences to illustrate and refute these perceived dangers. First, when I was training for a marathon under the Florida sun, I made the mistake of drinking only water and a sport drink which did not contain sodium. My hands swelled up like balloons. I called my mother, who brought me to the emergency room. They rapidly started IVs and measured my blood sodium, which was dangerously low. The medical term is dilutional hyponatremia, or low blood sodium levels caused by water dilution. I hadn't made any urine because there was little sodium to pull waste out of my bloodstream, and my main concern was not losing kidney function. My mind was already clouding over and, if my sodium levels had been any lower, I would have had a seizure. At the end of my stay, the doctor explained, "We see a lot of this here for Northerners who aren't acclimated. Next time, drink Gatorade." I had taken in too much water without enough sodium. Drinking a sport drink with more sodium would have saved me a lot of grief. This would be an example of a rare situation where too much water is actually dangerous.

On another jogging outing, this time in the Northwoods, I was suddenly seized with excruciating, drop-to-the-ground pain below my lowest rib in my back. I was paralyzed with pain and completely alone in the middle of nowhere. I figured I had either a ruptured aneurysm and would die in a few moments, or I had a kidney stone. I limped and crawled back to our cabin, where my wife and friends drove me 20 miles over bumpy dirt roads to the local E.R. The doctor hesitated to give me a narcotic, even though I told him the diagnosis. It was an agonizing wait for my test results to return, but they proved that I had blood in my urine, consistent with the presence of a kidney stone. The stone finally passed—three weeks later! After X-rays, doctor bills, physical exams, and weeks of pain, my urologist simply said, "Joe, drink more water." I was surprised to learn that surgeons have the highest frequency of kidney stones among all professions because they routinely dehydrate themselves as they scrub in on three- to six-hour procedures.

As for the "dangers" of too much water, I believe that the only real danger is in extreme circumstances like my Florida marathon. In most cases, because our diets are high in sodium, problems like low blood sodium are not an issue. I urge you to drink plenty of water every day. I recommend drinking spring water or filtered water. Filtered water does not contain minerals, while spring water does. Drinking lots of water has many important benefits beyond the reduced risk of kidney stones. Many studies show that people who drink less water have higher rates of bladder cancer, the fourth most common cancer in the United States. Perhaps the cancer-causing agents are more concentrated in the urine and soak into the bladder wall, causing cells to transition into a precancerous state. Studies have also shown that staying hydrated reduces the frequency of headaches, helps with weight loss, supports the immune system, and improves mental and physical performance.

## SKIN CARE

The skin is the largest organ of the body. It requires more attention than other organs because it's where we meet the world. It is exposed to all manner of stresses and insults.

Skin regenerates. We slough off skin cells constantly as they are replaced from our deeper skin layers, pushing up to the surface. Keeping this in mind, any topical (surface) attention, such as skin creams, lotions, or moisturizers, needs to be applied regularly. The goal is to keep those surface skin cells supple and moist.

Moisture also comes to the skin from inside the body. Good skin care also includes drinking a lot of water. Coffee, tea, and soda all contain water, but because of other chemicals they contain, they don't count as much toward your daily water need of around a half gallon.

Our skin constantly emits water through perspiration. During dry times of the year or in dry places, our skin actually has a direct fluid loss. We also lose water from our bodies from our lungs when we breathe. Those sources, in addition to our kidney output, equal at least half a gallon of water a day. To help your skin stay moist, be sure it has a reservoir of water to draw on from your daily routine.

Another important basic of skin care is to be conscious of what you put on your skin. Harsh chemicals may be great to clean the bathtub, but they don't do anything positive for your skin. When you're cleaning, wear rubber gloves.

Swimming in chlorinated pools or soaking in a chlorinated hot tub gives your skin a workout. When you're done and have showered with a gentle liquid soap, be certain to use a good body moisturizer to keep your skin healthy.

Skin-care science is making huge advances with anti-aging and anti-wrinkle products as well as targeted moisturizers for different types of skin and different areas of the body. *Alphahydroxy acids* (AHA), once limited to medical use, have crossed over into the commercial market. Products containing AHA make remarkable changes in the skin and seem to reduce tiny wrinkles.

Many skin care companies sell their products through upscale stores or on the Internet. As with diet and exercise, skin care needs are very individual. What you see and feel when you use a product is the best research you can do. You may sample many skin products in specialty or upscale department stores to find those which work best for you. Personally I use a combination of vitamin C and E, any available hydroxy acid gel, the moisturizing and nourishing plant-based natural skin care products from **Aveda** (developed by Horst Rechelbacher), and last but not least a broad-spectrum sunscreen.

Earlier in this book you read about medical interventions for skin care, but those are beyond the basics. Your plastic surgeon can refer you to an aesthetician to provide regular, in-depth skin care to keep your biggest organ glowing and restored.

The combination of a healthy diet, exercise, and daily skin care is an unbeatable combination whether or not your plan includes cosmetic surgery. We all have control over these three elements of beauty and health. The goal is not to remain twenty-eight forever, but rather to feel the youngest, healthiest, fittest, and most beautiful we can be at every age.

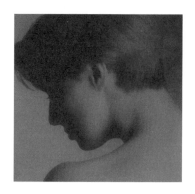

*chapter 13*

# THE ZONE DIET

"The benefits of plastic surgery can become
dramatically enhanced by paying careful attention
to the diet, and specifically *The Zone Diet.*"

– Dr. Barry Sears

*A*s a gift, I give patients who are worried about their weight a book called *A Week in the Zone* by Dr. Barry Sears. Dr. Sears used scientific research to develop *The Zone Diet*. The original *Zone* books were published for cardiologists. They can be difficult to understand, and the calculations needed can be threatening. The concise *A Week in the Zone* answers the most frequently asked questions, provides a simple method for choosing food, and gives a list of resources. Dr. Sears' website, **www.drsears.com**, has lots of good information. Hundreds of frequently asked questions are answered and hints, which can be adapted to your specific needs as you begin your new life in *The Zone*, are posted.

Dr. Sears views food—particularly carbohydrates—as medicine. His dietary plan looks at food in terms of how it affects the body's insulin production and, ultimately, energy production and fat storage. The type of food we eat sends our insulin up and our blood sugar down, our estrogen up and our growth hormones down.

## CARBS ARE THE CULPRITS

As I mentioned in Chapter 8 on *Liposuction*, some authorities believe we are born with only so many fat cells. Fat is stored in these cells, so when a person isn't eating, the cells shrink. When we eat more calories, the cells expand. In fact, according to Dr. Sears, once the existing fat cells fill completely, they give a signal for your body to **make even more fat cells**. He states that fat cells can grow more fat cells. This is the downside of the yo-yo diet syndrome. **You gain weight** (**and more fat cells**), then lose weight. Your fat cells shrink with weight loss, but the total number of fat cells remains increased.

In *The Zone* lifestyle, the quantity of food is less important than the quality of the food we eat. Yes, that's right. For years I thought it was just calories, but some calories are stored more efficiently than others. Even with severe calorie restriction, you can still gain weight on a high carbohydrate diet. Remember, it's your hormones that make your body store fat more or less efficiently.

Carbohydrates are the culprit in driving insulin levels up and making the body an efficient fat-storage machine. That's the key to the whole ball game. Actually eating pure fat, such as a teaspoon of virgin olive oil, doesn't affect insulin levels at all. The popular low-carb Atkins Diet has the right idea. Dr. Atkins' big push was exclusively toward low carbohydrates. Forget about eating bacon and eggs for breakfast and high-fat foods all day. Let that go. Just think about low carbohydrates. That's what helped his patients consistently lose weight.

One of the biggest issues with carbohydrates is how fast they're absorbed into your bloodstream. The glycemic index shows how fast carbohydrates are broken down into sugar and absorbed. Tables have been made up to show the differences between carbohydrate foods. Pure table sugar is assigned a number, and then other foods are compared to that. The glycemic load gives a person an idea of the body's physiological response to the type and amount of carbohydrate consumed.

The more carbohydrates you eat, the more insulin you produce. The more insulin you produce, the fatter you become, according to Dr. Sears. Think of it. How do farmers fatten cattle? On low-fat grain, which ups their insulin and causes the cattle to gain weight. Rice and grains are carbohydrates that cause insulin to spike more than others foods. Humans only have eaten grains for about the past eight thousand years, and our bodies aren't really put together to handle them very well, according to Dr. Sears' theory.

Promoters of a low-fat, high-carbohydrate diet are finding that heart attack rates are actually increased in patients on such strict diets. The American Heart Association is reevaluating standards in this area and recommendations have been made to maintain a diet more like *The Zone Diet*.

Most of the time when I mention *The Zone* to patients, they say, "Oh, I've heard of that. It's that high protein diet." In some ways this is true. American diets are loaded with fat and carbohydrates. *The Zone* is really a balanced diet. It includes proteins, carbohydrates, and fat—but they are always eaten together. So in a sense, there is more protein than the normal diet, but it's not a high-protein diet at all. In fact, the grams of carbohydrates are higher than the grams of protein in a *Zone* meal. Protein acts like the brakes on a car. It keeps the glycemic load from going into your blood stream too rapidly and firing up your insulin. How well you control your insulin level determines when you will become hungry.

It's well documented in the research literature that fish oils reduce the rate of heart attacks. Look at the Eskimos, who eat a lot of fat and fish oil. Heart disease and stroke are almost unheard of in their culture. The health benefits of high dose, pharmaceutical-grade fish oil also have been seen in *Zone Diet* research. This is one of the best sources of fat because it's so effective against inflammation. Seafood is loaded with this good fat. The best sources come from fish, such as salmon, mackerel, or sardines. Fish oils also fight the types of diseases that cause inflammation in our bodies, including arthritis, fibromyalgia, even multiple sclerosis.

Many authorities, including myself, believe the cholesterol deposited inside arteries is part of an inflammatory process. A C-reactive protein is a nonspecific marker of inflammation. People with CRP in higher concentrations are more likely to have strokes, heart attacks, and vessel diseases. In women, the concentrations are also affected by hormone status. Following *The Zone Diet* will help prevent inflammation.

## ZONE MEALS

Eating in *The Zone* involves three meals and two snacks every day. In practical terms, you can divide your meal plate into three sections. Fill one-third with a low-fat protein. This should be about the size and thickness of the palm of your hand. Then Dr. Sears recommends super-sizing the remainder of your meal with vegetables and fruits. Finally, you can add a dash of heart healthy fat, such as olive oil, avocado, or slivered almonds. *The Zone Diet* matches the way humans are genetically programmed to eat; low-fat protein, fruits and vegetables, and a small amount of monounsaturated fat.

In *The Zone*, you should eat within one hour of waking up. Eat every four to five hours whether you're hungry or not to keep insulin levels constant. Lack of hunger or cravings for sweets, along with good mental clarity, are indications you're in *The Zone*. Think of the food you eat as a healthy drug. When you take a medication, you take it once a day or at given intervals. A *Zone* meal should keep you in *The Zone* for four to five hours, whereas a *Zone* snack should be good for about two to two-and-a-half hours. If you're hungry two hours after eating a meal, you know your insulin level spiked.

After about five days, you should notice a decrease in hunger, along with greater mental clarity, greater physical performance, and less fatigue. *The Zone Diet* doesn't result in rapid weight loss, but eventually you should reach your goal. Depending on how much you exercise, you will lose between one to one-and-a-half pounds per week. You'll notice your clothes fit better after a couple of weeks.

If you are not overweight, you should eat in *The Zone* anyway. Remember, *The Zone* isn't a diet, it's a lifestyle. On that same note, food isn't food, it's a healthy drug. It is important to keep your insulin levels balanced whether you are overweight or not.

*The Zone Diet* has been purported to fight heart disease, diabetes, arthritis, fatigue, depression, cancer, hormone-related mood changes, multiple sclerosis, fibromyalgia, and myriad disorders related to the enigmatic inflammatory process.

You don't have to be obsessive about it. Just do the best you can. Even if you fall off the wagon once in a while, the results will be the same in the long run. Simply go back into *The Zone* the next time you eat, and I believe you'll feel healthier, have more energy, and be more alert.

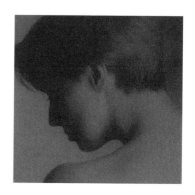

*chapter 14*

# FREQUENTLY ASKED

# QUESTIONS

"There's no such thing as a stupid question."

– Anonymous

## IS PLASTIC SURGERY RIGHT FOR ME?

**What is plastic surgery?**

The Greek word *plasticos* means "to shape, mold, or form." Plastic surgery can restore a patient with a serious deformity to a more "normal" appearance, but it can also help to rebuild someone's self-esteem.

**Who should read this book?**

Busy people who want a quick, readable source of information on cosmetic surgery should read this book. This guide is a friendly reference with essential tidbits of information to help you make an informed decision about cosmetic surgery.

**Who chooses plastic surgery?**

According to the most recent statistics from the American Society of Aesthetic Plastic Surgery (ASAPS), the number of cosmetic surgeries jumped 465 percent from 1997 to 2004. Nearly 11.9 million cosmetic procedures were performed in 2004 alone. Statistics indicate 92 percent of patients were women and eight percent were men.

Forty-five percent of people having cosmetic procedures were between the ages of 35 and 50; 24 percent were between the ages of 19 to 34; 22 percent were people aged from 51 to 64. People aged above 65 and below 18 had the least amount of plastic surgery, six percent and three percent respectively. Among U.S. citizens, 55 percent of women and 54 percent of men say they approve of cosmetic surgery.

**Is it unhealthy for people to be unhappy with the way they look?**

I don't believe it is. I believe the goal of plastic surgery should not be to change someone's basic appearance, but to prevent one from looking older than necessary, to enhance body image, and to elevate self-esteem. Plastic surgery is similar to living in a beautiful older home. It's only beautiful if it's kept in good repair. If the porch sags, I fix it. Why treat your body with less care?

**Is plastic surgery frivolous?**

I don't think so. I've seen many patients energized by a rejuvenating surgical procedure. My goal is to help people be happy with their appearance and improve how they feel about themselves.

### Is plastic surgery risky?

Plastic surgery isn't dieting, exercise, or other forms of self-improvement. It does expose you to a certain degree of health risk and is no different from any other kind of operation in that respect. Having said that, the vast majority of cosmetic procedures have a low rate of complications. Remember, you may end up dissatisfied with the result and need revisional surgery. Problems occur because doctors aren't able to read their patients' minds. Ideas of beauty are intangible and a patient's concept of larger, smaller, or prettier may not be the same as the surgeon's.

If you are ambivalent about plastic surgery, then come back for a second visit or call your surgeon on the phone to review the situation as many times as you need to.

### How can I research plastic surgery?

One of the best ways to research is on the Internet. For example, patients who consult me about breast augmentation should review photographs of rippling, asymmetry, visible contour problems, and size issues. People who use the Internet are the most informed consumers I encounter in my practice.

### Where can I look for information online?

Gryskiewicz Twin Cities Cosmetic Surgery's website:
www.tcplasticsurgery.com

Other sources:
www.implantinfo.com
www.lookingyourbest.com
www.plasticsurgery.org
www.makemeheal.com
www.breastdrs.com
www.surgery.org
www.breastimplantsafety.com

### When shouldn't I contemplate plastic surgery?

Just because you've decided to have plastic surgery doesn't mean you should. For every reason to have cosmetic surgery, there are reasons not to. Some good reasons not to have plastic surgery include:

· To please anyone other than yourself.
· As a reaction to a midlife crisis.
· As a reaction to a life-changing event, such as a death or divorce.
· If you suffer from ongoing depression.
· If you have any major health problems.
· To try to land "Mr. Wonderful" or "Ms. Fabulous."
· To just "be happy."

If you're a perfectionist and want guaranteed results, if you have multiple preoperative consultations and still feel indecisive, or if your intuition simply tells you "no," then you should also avoid cosmetic surgery. In addition, if you are ambivalent about cosmetic surgery, then make a list of questions you wish to ask your surgeon and ask him or her to explain each query in detail.

## UNDERSTANDING MEDICAL TITLES, CERTIFICATIONS, QUALIFICATIONS, AND SPECIALTIES

### What qualifications should I look for in a surgeon?

You need to look for three different qualifications in a surgeon: a medical degree (M.D.), board certification, and a state license. An M.D. requires four years of full-time study at a university. After receiving a medical degree most physicians enroll in a residency program, which allows them to specialize in a particular area. To become a plastic surgeon, the physician must complete a minimum of five years of surgical training after medical school, including a plastic surgery residency program, before passing an examination to become board certified.

Look for a plastic surgeon certified by the American Board of Plastic Surgery, as this is the only board approved by the American Board of Medical Specialties and the American Medical Association Council on Medical Education for certifying physicians in plastic surgery. This training encompasses both reconstructive and cosmetic surgery procedures for the face and body. Third, a state license must be obtained from the state in which the physician wants to practice.

**What should I look out for? And what is the difference between a cosmetic and a plastic surgeon?**

Currently any licensed physician is legally allowed to perform cosmetic surgery procedures. In fact, if you have an M.D. after your name you could even conduct brain surgery, whether you have surgical training or not! Luckily there are some structures in place to prevent a physician from doing this—insurance companies will not allow a surgeon on their rosters unless they are board certified, and hospitals restrict privileges unless appropriate training can be documented.

Here is a warning: A lot of cosmetic surgery is done in private offices or in surgery centers, so people can call themselves "cosmetic surgeons." Although these surgeons lack hospital privileges, the name "cosmetic surgeon" lends a measure of credibility in the professional community. To avoid disappointment or an unprofessional result, make sure the doctor you choose is a board-certified plastic surgeon and make sure she or he is certified by the American Board of Plastic Surgery (ABPS).

Anyone can create a board and claim to be certified by it. Look out for such boards as The American Board of Cosmetic Surgery, or any other board that is not recognized by The American Board of Medical Specialties. As a consumer, your best choice is to choose an ABPS-certified plastic surgeon with a particular interest in cosmetic surgery. In addition to board certification, the plastic surgeon will also probably belong to the American Society of Plastic Surgeons (ASPS). Almost all board-certified plastic surgeons belong to the ASPS.

**What is a skimmer?**

"Skimmers" are physicians without plastic-surgery training who are performing cosmetic procedures as a way to boost their income. They don't want to put in the hours of training to become a plastic surgeon, yet they "skim" the profits off this potentially lucrative branch of cosmetic surgery.

**What really matters with cosmetic surgery?**

What really matters is the patients' rights and safety. Patients have the right to know the full nature and extent of their doctor's formal training and to choose any physician they wish. I suggest patients discuss the procedure with their surgeon and ask to see before and after photographs of previous patients to help ascertain whether they will be happy with the result. If you do not like the results, or if you do not feel comfortable with your chosen surgeon, then you should go elsewhere.

**Where can I check a surgeon's credentials?**

There are four main ways to validate your surgeon's credentials:

- The American Society for Aesthetic Plastic Surgery (ASAPS) **888-ASAPS-11**. Their website is: **www.surgery.org**.
- The American Society of Plastic Surgeons (ASPS) **www.plasticsurgery.org**.
- The American Board of Medical Specialists (ABMS) at **www.abms.org**.
- Your state's Medical Board at **www.mhsource.com/resource/board.html**.

**What are the requirements for election to the American Society of Aesthetic Plastic Surgery (ASAPS)?**

Election to ASAPS involves:

- Certification by the American Board of Plastic Surgery.
- A minimum of three years active practice following board certification.
- A surgical case list demonstrating an extensive number of cosmetic procedures.
- Documented continuing medical education credits in cosmetic surgery for 36 months prior to the application.
- Sponsorship by two active members.
- Submission of current marketing and advertising materials for review.
- Adherence to the society's code of ethics for professional conduct.

## HOW TO CHOOSE A COSMETIC SURGEON: A FOOLPROOF METHOD

**How do I find an excellent cosmetic surgeon?**

- Familiarize yourself with the physician's qualifications, titles, and certifications (see immediately above).
- Use the Yellow Pages with discretion. Any physician can call himself or herself a plastic surgeon, so use the telephone book as a guide and not the basis of your research.
- Beware of false advertising. Never select a plastic surgeon on advertising alone.
- Do some online research.
- Learn as much as you can about the procedure you want.
- Ask for recommendations from acquaintances who have had plastic surgery.
- Consult your family doctor.

- Ask your hairdresser. You may not have thought of it but they are in an excellent position to evaluate how different facelift, brow-lift, and eyelid scars are hidden.
- Ask for pertinent references (you have the right to do this). Most doctors keep a patient referral list of people who are happy to discuss their cosmetic procedure.
- Beware of the hype. Being quoted in a popular magazine, appearing on television, or speaking on radio does not guarantee a surgeon's qualifications.
- Check with professional organizations. Call the ASPS's physician-referral service to receive a list of five members who practice in your area. Also call the ABPS to find out whether the surgeon you have in your mind is board certified. The ASAPS can also help you locate surgeons in your area.
- Ask the specialty of the surgeon you have in mind.
- Call your state's medical board to check on your doctor.
- Meet with different doctors.
- Choose a surgeon you both trust and feel confident with.

## What happens in the initial consultation?

A nurse usually begins the consultation by taking the patient to the examination room and showing them a video about the particular procedure they are interested in. After this, I have a conversation with the patient, assess whether he or she is a suitable candidate for the type of procedure, and discuss the procedure in detail.

## What happens at the end of the initial consultation?

Patients are seen in my private office, and in this calm setting I give a little "surgery sermon" which encompasses the potential risks, limitations, and benefits of the procedure, as they apply to the patient. We also talk about the cost and any other issues or questions the person has. From a patient's point of view, you should be evaluating your potential surgeon and asking yourself if you feel comfortable with the surgeon, and making sure you are able to interact with your doctor.

## What are some good questions to ask my cosmetic surgeon?
- Ask where the procedure will be performed. Will it be in a hospital, at a private surgery center, or in a same-day facility? If the doctor operates a same-day surgery or office-based facility, ask if it's accredited.

- Ask about your doctor's hospital privileges.
- Ask who will administer the anesthesia and who is ultimately responsibility for the anesthesia—the surgeon or the anesthesiologist.
- Ask about the surgeon's experience in performing the procedure.
- Ask to see before and after photographs.
- Ask about the policy on surgical revisions, because a small number of cases require revisions to achieve the desired result.
- Ask what risks the procedure has in relation to your medical history.
- Ask what kind of result is realistic for you to expect.
- Ask about the expected recovery time for your particular procedure.

## HOW TO BE A TERRIFIC PATIENT AND GET EVERYTHING YOU WANT FROM A PLASTIC SURGEON

### Am I ready for plastic surgery?

Make sure you are 100 percent prepared for surgery, because preoperative ambivalence directly correlates to postoperative dissatisfaction. If you don't trust your surgeon, then don't have the procedure. If your expectations are realistic, then you should be pleased with the results, no matter how subtle or dramatic they are.

### How accurate is computer imaging?

Many cosmetic surgeons employ computer-imaging technology to help patients make up their mind about the procedure. These techniques are an excellent way to make sure you and your doctor are on the same wavelength. However, you must understand a photo is not a guarantee of an exact outcome.

### What are some dos and don'ts in the consultation process?
- *Do* be specific. It is vital to communicate honestly with your doctor about your needs and to be assertive about what you want.
- *Don't* let your partner make decisions about your procedure. You should be doing this for you, not for anybody else.
- *Do* give your doctor the benefit of the doubt. If you have done your research and she or he is well qualified, then listen to what the doctor says. If the doctor is late to the appointment and you have to wait, be patient. Doctors are busy people and emergencies arise. Please give the doctor a second chance.

- *Don't* interrupt. Wait for your doctor to ask if you have any questions and then go over your list.
- *Do* take no for an answer. If your surgeon refuses to operate on you, listen to the reason why. You can always get a second opinion, but be wary of choosing a surgeon who puts his or her best interest ahead of yours.
- *Don't* lie about smoking. It could seriously jeopardize the outcome of your operation.
- *Do* be honest when filling out your medical history.

**Are there risks of surgical complication?**

With any surgery there are risks, however the percentage of complications in cosmetic procedures is very low as long as the following safeguards are in place:
- The case is not prolonged.
- Excessive volume is not being removed.
- The medical facility is accredited.
- The surgeon uses sterile technique.
- The surgeon has performed a preoperative analysis, a physical examination, and has a reputation for excellent technical execution of the procedure.
- The patient complies with preoperative precautions.
- The patient is truthful about the medical history.

**Will smoking affect the outcome of my procedure?**

Many surgeons, including myself, will not perform surgeries such as an abdominoplasty or facelift on patients who smoke. Discontinuing smoking is recommended for all surgeries and is essential for some, such as an abdominoplasty or facelift. Every time nicotine enters the body, blood supply is limited and the surgical area is jeopardized. For example, in a facelift, the skin can die and slough off. Patients should not lie about whether they smoke. The lie could seriously jeopardize the outcome.

Also, smoking directly affects the skin's ability to regenerate and rejuvenate itself. It promotes loss of elasticity, resulting in multiple, deep wrinkles.

**What are the costs involved?**

The costs of plastic surgery vary depending on the patient's needs and the extent and difficulty of the procedure. Financing for cosmetic procedures may be available. The cost of the surgery will include the surgeon's fees, fees from the surgical facility, and the cost of the anesthesia. Be sure to obtain the projected fees in writing. Other possible costs are the preoperative physical and blood work, pathology reports, postoperative medications, surgical garments, and private-duty nursing. Advance payment is usually required and is common practice nationally. Cosmetic surgery is not tax deductible.

**What are the risks involved in cosmetic surgery?**

ASAPS statistics indicate over 11 million cosmetic procedures are performed annually, and public concern about the safety of cosmetic surgery is increasing just as steadily. There are several risks involved in all cosmetic surgery procedures, and to reduce this risk patients should make sure they are operated on in an accredited facility. Possible risks include anesthesia allergy (although the chance is less than one in a million), fluid loss (which can result from long procedures), blood and fat clots, infection caused by unsterilized equipment, and shock.

**Will insurance cover the costs?**

No. Insurance doesn't cover cosmetic surgery, although some surgical procedures such as rhinoplasty to improve your breathing or breast reconstruction after a mastectomy, are a combination of cosmetic and reconstructive surgery, which is often covered by insurance. Fees for the reconstructive portion of a surgery cannot ethically be increased to cover any portion of the procedure. Insurance companies have reasonable and customary fees on which they base payments.

**How is payment made and what does the cost involve?**

Advance payment is usually required and is common practice nationally. Financing programs are available from the ASPS for people who do not want to delay the process because they cannot afford to pay in advance. Costs include all of the items listed above. Patients usually write one check to me and another to the surgery center. Be sure to obtain fees in writing.

## DOCTOR AND PATIENT RELATIONSHIPS

**What is the appropriate doctor/patient relationship?**

It is common for patients to feel close to their surgeon. However, there are some guidelines to remember in regard to this relationship. Remember, in reality you do not know your physician as a person. To take a relationship outside the clinical setting is not fair to either party involved.

**Is it normal to feel depressed after surgery?**

You may find you feel depressed in the week or so following surgery. This is a normal reaction to the anesthesia and to the changes your body has undergone. Just ride it out and try not to worry about it too much. You will feel better soon.

**What are the different types of anesthesia?**

Your procedure will be done under local, sedation, or general anesthesia.

*Local*—with or without sedation if small procedures are involved, a local anesthetic can be used to numb the area. You may be given a mild sedative to help you relax. This is referred to as *intravenous sedation* or *monitored anesthesia.*

*Sedation*—comes in the form of intravenous sedation. A catheter is inserted into the vein and a continuous flow of anesthetic is delivered. You're in a twilight sleep when this method is used.

*General*—in this case you will be unconscious throughout the procedure and usually have a breathing tube inserted for its duration.

## BREAST SURGERIES

### Breast Augmentation

**At what age do most women receive a breast augmentation?**

Breast augmentation is the most popular cosmetic procedure among women. The average age of women seeking this procedure is around 32, however they range from 18 to their 60s. The patient is likely to have had children and breastfed one of them before wanting breast augmentation surgery.

**What can a breast augmentation do?**
- Enhance breast size and shape.
- Restore breast volume.
- Help clothes and swimwear fit better.
- Correct asymmetries and differences in breast size.
- Reconstruct breasts after a mastectomy performed for cancer or premalignant conditions.

## What size should I choose?

This is the big question and is a hard question to answer. I measure a patient's rib cage, breast fold, tissue thickness, breast width and even the distance of the nipple and areola to the belly button and shoulders during my examination to ascertain how the woman will carry the size of the implant. My staff and I try to be exceptionally thorough in this very personal portion of the consult. Our patients benefit from the details we put into this important question. We extensively discuss the trade-offs of larger versus smaller implants.

## What type of implant should I choose?

I use both silicone and saline implants. Silicone gel implants look more natural and feel softer. Studies show silicone implants do not increase the incidence of disease or the chances of developing breast or other cancers. Silicone and saline implants come in various shapes: round, teardrop and oval. I prefer a standard round implant although the pros and cons of each shape and type should be discussed with your surgeon.

## What does the breast augmentation procedure involve?

I favor placing the implant under the chest muscle, because my radiology colleagues think this position interferes less with the detection of breast cancer. Not all surgeons agree on this, but I prefer to err on the side of caution. Submuscular placement helps to avoid visible rippling. The muscle adds a thicker cover over the implant shell except for the lower, outside portion of the breast where wrinkling is most common. The alternative is to place the implant on top of the muscle. The implants can be inserted through incisions in the armpit, around the areola, in the crease of the base of the breast, or even through the belly button. I let the woman decide on the location of her incision, and most women choose the armpit incision because they don't want to scar their breasts.

## What needs to be done before the operation?

Before surgery I use a marker to draw the incisions and the entire surgical plan on the patient's chest. The plan includes the type of incision, implant size on each side, placement of the implant with respect to the nipple location and placement toward the inside or the outside of the breastbone. Patients take three Hibiclens (chlorhexidene) showers the night before surgery, because washing the chest and armpits helps prevent infection. During the surgery an intravenous antibiotic kills specific germs that are implicated in capsular contracture. Surgery is done on a same-day basis and takes one hour to complete.

### How long is the recovery time?

With modern breast augmentation procedures, if patients have surgery on Friday, then they can return to work on Monday. Pain medication is prescribed to alleviate any discomfort, and I also prescribe a muscle relaxant and anti-nausea medication. Patients do not have to take antibiotic pills after surgery.

### What is dual-plane breast augmentation?

Seventeen percent of my augmentations are done with a dual-plane or "internal lift" approach to lift breast tissue, elevate the nipple-areola complex, and to release a tight breast crease. This is technically a breast enlargement procedure. The technique avoids the more extensive scars of an external "classic" lift and can be especially useful in fixing early sagging.

### What is rapid-recovery breast augmentation?

I specialize in rapid-recovery breast augmentation, also known as the "no touch technique." It is a surgical procedure that uses special instruments and techniques to minimize tissue damage and avoid touching the ribs. It causes far less trauma to surrounding tissue than traditional approaches, and it dramatically reduces pain, suffering, and recovery time. In my experience, 95 percent of women interviewed after the procedure returned to normal daily activities within 24 hours. Medical references are available. Individual results vary.

### What happens after rapid-recovery breast augmentation?

There are three very important things to do after surgery:
- Get your arms over your head, and do three arm raises every hour before going to bed.
- Don't baby your breasts, because you can't rupture or rip open your stitches.
- Lie on your breasts for 15 minutes every day starting on the evening of your surgery. Not only will you feel better but you will also lessen the risk of developing scar tissue around the implant.

### Will breast implants affect the detection of breast cancer?

An implant will impair the accuracy of a mammogram to some extent. You should notify the technician about the implants when having a mammography so additional views can be taken to examine the breast tissue more effectively.

## What are the risks and limitations of breast augmentation surgery?

Implants can rupture. A rupture is usually caused by a small pinpoint leak that can develop on the implant's edge. Implants need to be replaced if they rupture. Implants can become infected, although this is rare. Nipple numbness occurs in about three percent of cases. Other complications include capsular contracture, visible wrinkling, and folds.

### Breast Lift or Mastopexy

## What is a breast lift?

A breast lift, otherwise known as a *mastopexy*, is a procedure to elevate the nipple-areola complex and to tighten the skin envelope. When breast sag is severe, additional incisions and skin removal may be required.

## When do I need a mastopexy?

When the nipple is well below the breast crease a mastopexy is required. The procedure is usually performed following childbirth or after breastfeeding. Extremely large, heavy breasts tend to sag after a mastopexy so women with these may not be the best candidates for the procedure. Ideal candidates are women with moderate-sized breasts who are finished having children. Mastopexy can be personally tailored to suit the individual.

## What are some points to consider when contemplating a mastopexy?

These points need consideration:
- If your breasts differ markedly, do you want a lift and a reduction on the larger side?
- How much scarring can you tolerate?
- Determine which procedure will give you the most improvement with the least scarring.
- Do you want a smaller areola?
- Are you planning to have children? And would you like to breastfeed them?

## What is the most important element in patient satisfaction?

Have realistic expectations. Results are not permanent. Gravity, weight fluctuations, and aging take their toll on your breasts again.

## What does the mastopexy or breast lift procedure involve?

A mastopexy is a same-day procedure usually done under general anesthesia but occasionally under intravenous sedation if limited incisions are used. The procedure takes about one and a half hours to three and a half hours to perform. Depending on the level of the nipple and the amount of excess skin, incisions can range from a small crescent above the areola to the doughnut and the classic anchor incision pattern.

A mastopexy is a three-dimensional operation. If it is combined with a breast augmentation, then be prepared to experience some differences from one side to the other. Scarring is considerable, even in a "minimal incision" procedure.

## What happens after surgery?

The breasts will be bruised and swollen after surgery. Swelling will be minimal to moderate and will last several weeks. A moderate level of pain should be expected and pain medication will be prescribed. Immediately after surgery the patient may wear an elastic wrap or a surgical support bra with gauze bandages. The patient must wear a good support bra around the clock for three to four weeks. Vigorous exercise should be avoided, as should sleeping on your stomach. If massive swelling appears on one side, or fever, redness, or unusual draining is experienced, you should consult your surgeon immediately.

## What is the recovery time?

Lifting anything above your head should be avoided for at least four weeks after a breast lift. Engaging in strenuous activities should be avoided for the same period of time.

## What are the risks and limitations involved in a mastopexy?

Numbness may occur in the nipple area or in scattered areas of breast skin. Bleeding can occur, even to the degree that a secondary drainage procedure may become necessary. In rare cases mastopexy procedures could affect your ability to breast-feed. Many surgeons avoid performing a mastopexy until a woman has finished childbearing because pregnancy tends to stretch the breast skin. Mastopexy leaves noticeable scars, although these can be covered by your bra or bathing suit.

### Breast Reconstruction

### What is a breast reconstruction?

Awareness of the physical and psychological benefits of breast-reconstruction surgery is growing. New surgical options are available, and advances in the field are helping surgeons create softer, more sensitive, and natural-looking breasts. However fewer women are choosing to have "immediate reconstruction" at the time of a mastectomy.

### Will a breast reconstruction increase the risk of breast cancer recurrence?

No. There is no evidence to suggest this. If your oncologist recommends a mastectomy and you plan to have a reconstruction, ask for a referral to a plastic surgeon. In most cases breast reconstruction is covered by insurance.

### Breast Reduction

### What is a breast reduction?

Women with heavy breasts may suffer from a skeletal imbalance that contributes to back, neck, and shoulder pain. Some also experience numbness in their hands and breathing problems due to nerve compression as their breasts pull down on their shoulders. The goal of a breast reduction is to relieve these symptoms. The surgery is primarily done for medical reasons, but appearance can be enhanced as well. A breast reduction, also known as a reduction mammoplasty, involves removing excess fat, breast tissue, and skin. It is similar to a mastopexy, except that volume is removed as well as excess skin.

### Does insurance cover a breast reduction procedure?

Insurance may cover breast reduction for some women, however this usually depends on a special formula depending on the patient's breast size, body type, symptoms, and also their body weight, height, and how much your surgeon estimates will be removed. Usually a pound from each breast is needed for insurance coverage.

### What happens in a breast reduction procedure?

Breast reductions are usually done as same-day surgery. The procedure is performed under general anesthesia and lasts for two to three hours. Techniques vary. Before you decide on a technique, request to see photos of your surgeon's prior patients to help you understand what the scars will look like. The most common procedure involves an anchor-shaped scar pattern. The incision surrounds the areola, proceeds down the breast's center and ends along the breast crease. Surrounding breast and subcutaneous tissue is removed, along with excess skin, and the nipple and areola are raised to the level of the natural breast crease. Skin is folded around the central breast tissue to form a new breast shape. Liposuction may be used to remove the excess roll on the side of the breast. If the breasts are very large or the nipple is very low, your surgeon may choose to remove the nipple and graft it higher. If this is done, nipple sensation will be lost.

## What happens after surgery?

Patients will usually wear a support bra day and night for the first month, and sometimes drains will be used for a few days. Breasts generally remain bruised and swollen for a week or two.

## What are the risks and limitations of a breast reduction?

Numbness in the nipple or breast skin can occur and bleeding may occur which will require a secondary drainage procedure. Infection and separation of incisions in high-tension areas are also possible and a small portion of skin may die. Scarring will occur, although clothing will hide this.

## Can I breast-feed after a breast reduction?

Most women are able to breast-feed after surgery, but this can't be guaranteed.


# RHINOPLASTY, FACELIFTS, AND OTHER FACIAL PROBLEMS

## Rhinoplasty

## What is rhinoplasty or nose reshaping?

*Rhino* means *nose* and *plasty* means *to shape, mold, or form*. Rhinoplasty accounted for about two percent of all cosmetic surgery procedures in 2004. Many plastic surgeons feel rhinoplasty is the most artistic and difficult cosmetic surgical procedure. I agree, because the surgeon makes three-dimensional changes which instantly alter other areas of the nose.

### How important is the preoperative analysis in rhinoplasty?

Accurate preoperative analysis is 50 percent of the outcome. I encourage my patients to bring in photographs of how they envision the results. Only a limited number of experts specialize in rhinoplasty, so do your homework.

### What is involved in the procedure?

Rhinoplasty is done on a same-day basis. I prefer to use general anesthesia because there tends to be bleeding in the back of the throat, and this may be a problem with a semi-conscious patient. Ultimately, however, I tend to let the patient decide what anesthesia they would like. There are various techniques, depending on the anticipated outcome.

### Will I need to have any post-procedure touch-ups?

Because rhinoplasty is a complicated procedure and the nose swells during the operation, there is a chance you may need to have some post-surgery touch-ups. About 15 percent of rhinoplasty operations require touch-up procedures.

### What happens after rhinoplasty surgery?

At the conclusion of the procedure a long-acting numbing agent is used to ensure the patient leaves the surgery center pain-free. A splint is usually placed on the nose for one week. The nose will be noticeably swollen for several days, and shouldn't be blown. Half of rhinoplasty patients have some bruising. It may take up to a year before all traces of swelling disappear, but the nose will definitely look better by the time the splint comes off after surgery.

### What are the risks and limitations of rhinoplasty?

The biggest limitation with rhinoplasty is thick skin, because this is difficult to shrink and conform to the underlying framework of the procedure. A surgeon can only do so much with a large nose if the skin won't contract. Risks include infection, postoperative nose bleeds, numbness, swelling, possible collapse of the nose, external scarring, fullness, residual deformity, and holes inside the septal area of the nose.

### Facelift

### Why do people need facelifts?

Facelift procedures directly counteract the aging effects of gravity. In a matter of hours the clock is turned back and the patient's profile is transformed.

### Am I a candidate for a facelift?

The best candidate for a facelift has a face and neck that has begun to sag, good skin elasticity, and strong, well-defined bone structure. A person having a facelift will look seven to 10 years younger on average. The result of a facelift is permanent, but you will continue to age normally. This means you will look better at any given age than if you had not undergone the procedure.

### How do I avoid an "extreme" facelift?

The best way to avoid the "extreme" facelift—the kind we see on the overly taut skin of Hollywood stars—is to see a skilled practitioner. Ask to look at patient photographs; look at the results. If the faces appear overdrawn and tight, then seek your surgery elsewhere. Some signs that indicate a bad facelift include: tension lines, skin pleats, a distorted mouth, hairless scalp incisions, sideburns displaced upwards, and attached earlobes or "pixie ears."

### What does the facelift procedure involve?

Facelifts usually involve elevating the skin over the facial area, pulling it upwards, removing the excess and closing the incisions. Current practice now involves extensive work on the deeper facial structures. Discuss the type of facelift approach your surgeon plans to use, and be sure to find a surgeon with plenty of training and experience. The procedure generally takes several hours to perform and incisions begin above the hairline at the temples, extend down the natural line in front of the ear and continue behind the earlobe to the lower scalp. Skin is separated from fat and muscle below, and those tissues are trimmed, suctioned, incised, and tightened as needed.

### Can I have neck liposuction without a facelift?

Neck liposuction without a facelift is a reasonable alternative for some patients who are unwilling to undergo a facelift. Localized fullness in the middle of the neck with good overlying skin tone are usually the best indicators of a good outcome.

### What is a minimal incision facelift?

Also known as a short-scar facelift or mini-lift, this procedure is becoming very popular. It combines lipoplasty with less-invasive surgical procedures than those used in traditional facelifts. The best candidates for this type of surgery are younger patients with good skin elasticity.

### What happens after facelift surgery?

Discomfort after a facelift is usually minimal and can be managed with minor pain medication. Some facial numbness is normal and will disappear in a few weeks to months. To reduce swelling it is important to keep your head elevated in the weeks following surgery. Your face will feel bruised, puffy, and pale the day after surgery, but will improve as recovery progresses. Stitches will be removed after five days. Patients should take it easy in the weeks following a facelift. Strenuous exercise, sex, and heavy housework should be avoided, as should alcohol, steam baths, and saunas.

### What are the risks and limitations?

Complications include infection, hematoma, hairline elevation, baldness, skin loss or tissue death, delayed healing, skin numbness, facial weakness, and bad scarring. Very rarely have patients reported prolonged or permanent pain or uncomfortable sensations. Revisional surgery may be required in patients who are not happy with the result.

**Forehead Lift**

### What is a forehead lift?

A patient may want a forehead lift to correct drooping eyebrows. The procedure, also known as a brow lift, restores the eyelid area to a more youthful oval shape. If you look in the mirror, place your palms on your forehead on the outside edge of your eyes above your eyebrows, and gently raise the skin, you can get a feel for what a forehead lift can do for you.

### How is the forehead lift performed?

The classic approach to a forehead lift is to open the area through a curving scalp incision. Some forehead lifts are done through three or four small scalp incisions. An endoscope is inserted through one incision and instruments are inserted in others to lift the skin and muscle. At the same time, the surgeon removes or alters underlying tissues and the eyebrows may be lifted and secured into a higher position by sutures beneath the skin's surface.

### What happens after the forehead lift procedure?

Some numbness, incision discomfort, and mild swelling may be experienced after surgery. Pain at the incision site is usually minimal and can be managed through mild pain medication. Stitches and staples will be removed after one week and temporary fixation screws will be removed within two. Patients should take it easy for the week following surgery and most patients are back at work within a week. Vigorous physical activity should be avoided in the weeks following the procedure.

### What are the risks involved in a forehead lift?

Risks are minimal but include infection, bleeding, delayed healing, numbness, and temporary injury to the nerves that control eyebrow movement.

## Mid-face Lift

### What is a mid-face lift?

A mid-face lift elevates the cheeks and tissue from the lower eyelid down to the corners of the mouth. A traditional facelift, which deals with the neck and jaw line, doesn't lift tissue as well in this area.

### What happens in a mid-face lift?

Most surgeons make an incision below the lash line of the lower eyelid, and then go below the bone lining, also called the periosteum. This incision travels down over the cheekbone and eventually breaks through the periosteum into the soft tissue of the cheek fold. Pulling of the segment will raise the corner of the mouth. Another approach avoids the lower eyelid incision and uses an endoscope to guide an incision hidden behind the hairline along the side of the temple area and down into the cheek. In this approach a second incision is hidden in the mouth.

## Dermabrasion

### What is dermabrasion?

*Dermabrasion* involves the use of a high-speed rotating diamond brush on the facial skin, causing a controlled abrasion injury that eventually heals. This smoothes the skin to lessen acne scarring, fine lines and other irregularities. Dermabrasion can be an in-office procedure often done by dermatologists. Possible risks involve prolonged redness or itching, scarring and color changes.

## Blepharoplasty

### What is blepharoplasty or cosmetic eyelid surgery?

*Blepharoplasty* is a surgical procedure to remove excess skin and fat from the upper and lower eyelid. Drooping eyebrows and upper eyelids may impair your vision and diminish your appearance. This procedure can be done along with other cosmetic procedures and is highly individualized.

### Will blepharoplasty improve the condition of the skin surrounding my eyes?

Eyelid surgery will not remove fine smile lines, dark circles, or widespread crepey skin, which can be treated with peels, laser surgery, bleaching, and Botox injections.

### What does the blepharoplasty procedure involve?

Surgery is done on a same-day basis and may take anywhere from 30 minutes to two hours to complete. Patients are usually sedated and numbing drops are placed in each eye before local anesthesia is used to numb the surrounding area. There are two main approaches: internal and external. All scars are very inconspicuous.

### What should I do after a blepharoplasty procedure?

You should only experience mild discomfort following surgery. Pain medication will be prescribed. If you experience any pain or loss of vision, then notify your doctor immediately. The head should be elevated and vigorous activity avoided for one to two weeks. Bruising may be apparent for one to two weeks.

### What are the risks involved in a blepharoplasty procedure?

Patients should be in good health before they contemplate this surgery. A history of problems such as dry eyes, thyroid problems, or ongoing issues such as glaucoma, detached retina, or recent eye surgery should be evaluated before you proceed. There is a possibility that the upper eyelids may become "dog eared," meaning an area of fullness may develop at the end of the incision. Prolonged swelling may occur on one side of the face. The main risk with lower-lid procedures is the loss of muscle laxity that causes the lid to pull down.

### Chin Augmentation

#### What is a chin augmentation?

Aesthetic chin augmentation is a surgical procedure to reshape or increase the size of the chin. Patients who desire a balanced profile by extending the chin in relationship to the nose are suited to this procedure.

#### What does a chin augmentation procedure involve?

There are two basic approaches. In a genioplasty, an incision is made inside the mouth to gain access to the chin bone area. The lower portion of the bone is separated and is shifted forward and stabilized. When a modest degree of augmentation is required, the surgeon may recommend using a chin implant or prosthesis.

#### Will I be in pain after a chin augmentation?

There will be some soreness and discomfort, which can be easily controlled by pain medication. I advise a liquid diet for a week. Patients are generally up and around the same day and may return to work within a couple of days if they do not object to wearing a chin strap in public, which should be kept on for about a week.

#### What are the risks and limitations of a chin augmentation?

Risks include infection, bone reabsorption, numbness, displacement, extrusion, asymmetry, and bleeding. There is a small chance of chin drop or "witch's chin."

### Lip Augmentation

#### What is a surgical lip augmentation?

Surgical lip procedures offer a permanent alternative to collagen injections or other fillers. This can either be done through surgical manipulation or grafts.

#### What does the surgical lip augmentation procedure involve?

Grafts to enlarge the lips may be made up of skin, fat, or a combination of both, and may come from the patient's body or from a donor. The outer layer of any skin used is removed so that cysts do not form and the tissue is then placed in the lip area. The graft material acts as a framework and the body's tissue fills in the matrix. A surgical augmentation moves tissue from inside the mouth forward in a "W" pattern. This shifts mucosa toward the outside of the lip and rolls the lip outward, making it fuller in appearance. Lip enlargements may not be permanent and this is one reason for the different approaches.

### Fat Transfer

### What is a fat injection?

Also called *lipostructure infiltration*, a fat injection uses the patient's own body fat to fill folds and wrinkles. It involves harvesting fat from one body area, usually from the hips or stomach, and replacing it elsewhere, most commonly in the facial areas, especially the cheek folds and lips. The procedure is generally done under intravenous sedation or general anesthesia and takes about an hour. It can be combined with other surgeries and involves little pain.

### What are the risks and limitations of a fat transfer?

The main problem is that the body absorbs some of the fat. Further injections may be necessary and can be repeated every 6 to 12 months. Bleeding, infection, scarring, numbness, donor site problems, contour irregularities, and fullness are some of the risks of this procedure.

### Otoplasty

### What is otoplasty or cosmetic ear surgery?

The ear is 95 percent grown by the time a child is eight years old. Many children suffer psychological damage from being teased about their ears. Otoplasty for a congenital cup ear deformity can be performed on children before they begin school. The procedure is completed in an hour, with very little postoperative pain or discomfort. The risks include bleeding, infection, scarring, numbness, asymmetry, and loss of cartilage. Some bruising may occur.

### Cheek Implants

### What are cheek implants?

A cheek implant involves placing a prosthesis to give the patient a higher cheekbone. The approach can be through the mouth or through an incision made in the lower eyelid. I find it difficult to meet patient's expectations because patients complain the implants are either too big or too small, and asymmetries can be problematic because implants may shift. I have been dissuaded from this technique because of unhappy patients and other surgeons' opinions.

## Surface Work

### What surface work can be performed?

The appearance of the face can be enhanced with Botox, chemical peels, tissue fillers, and collagen injections. Botox is a temporary option that causes muscle paralysis, thereby reducing wrinkles. Chemical peels, which can be mild, moderate, or strong, can be used to rejuvenate facial skin and smooth facial wrinkles. Hyaluronic acid fillers are used to plump the tissue to improve fine lines, major wrinkles, cheek folds or lip size.

### What is laser skin resurfacing?

Laser resurfacing involves applying a beam or laser to the skin to alleviate wrinkles, acne or general scarring, age or brown spots, and sun-damaged skin. Best results are achieved with a full-face laser treatment because this uniformly stretches the skin throughout the facial area and produces a more homogenous color. This procedure can also be used to tighten the skin. Afterwards the patient's face will appear "scary." In an average treatment, crusts will form on the skin. Healing usually occurs from between five to 10 days, and the face may remain red for a couple of months, fading over the next year. Possible risks include infection, herpes outbreaks, postoperative scarring, permanent color changes to the skin, prolonged redness or itching, permanent patchy spots due to sun exposure, and failure of the surgery.

## BODY WORK

### Abdominoplasty

### What is an abdominoplasty or tummy tuck?

An *abdominoplasty* is a procedure designed to tighten the sagging abdominal muscles and to give the stomach area a flatter, smoother appearance. The procedure is commonly carried out on women after they have had children. All the sit-ups in the world will not bring the abdominal muscles back to normal if they have spread apart in pregnancy. Scars may be around the belly button, and extend from hip to hip running along the lower abdomen. An abdominoplasty is not a weight loss procedure. It benefits women who are in reasonably good shape but are plagued by an extensive fat deposit. In general, plastic surgeons defer abdominoplasty until after a woman has finished childbearing.

### What happens in an abdominoplasty procedure?

An abdominoplasty is not a simple operation. Your surgeon will have to determine the extent of the fat deposits and assess your skin and muscle tone. The procedure is generally carried out in a same-day surgery under a general anesthesia or heavy sedation. There are several different types of abdomino-plasty, depending on the patient's needs and anatomy. These include an endoscopic abdominoplasty, a modified or limited abdominoplasty, and a complete or classic abdominoplasty.

### How long does it take to recover from an abdominoplasty?

A patient's pain while recovering from an abdominoplasty can register about 8 on a scale of 1 to 10. Someone will need to help you around the house for a few days. Usually the abdomen is bruised for about three weeks and can feel slightly numb for several months. Drains will be required after you are discharged and elastic stockings should be worn to prevent blood clots in the legs. Heavy lifting (anything over 10 pounds) and vigorous exercise should be avoided for six to eight weeks. Patients can return to work within a week or two, as long as their job doesn't require any heavy lifting.

### What are the risks and complications associated with abdominoplasty?

Irregularity or asymmetry may persist and touch-up surgery may be required. A number of patients develop some fluid retention after their drains are removed. Bad scarring may be another untoward outcome. Blood clots can be avoided by being active after the procedure. The pubic line is elevated for a more youthful appearance, but in rare instances may be overly elevated after a tummy tuck.

#### Buttock Lift

### What is a buttock lift?

In some people the ligaments supporting the buttocks relax, either because of aging, weight loss, or pure genetics. In these cases a buttock lift removes a crescent of tissue from the uppermost aspect of each buttock, while the bottom portion is elevated. The procedure is usually accompanied by liposuction and in some cases the incisions can be extended all the way around the front of the body and combined with a tummy tuck for a 360-degree trunkoplasty.

### Liposuction

### What is liposuction?

*Liposuction* is the most common procedure performed by ABPS members. Liposuction removes deposits of subcutaneous fat over diverse areas of the body, from the face and neck, upper arms, trunk, abdomen, hips, buttocks, inner and outer thighs, knees, calves, and ankles.

### How does liposuction work?

The physiology is controversial. Some authorities believe a person is born with a certain number of fat cells. These cells grow and shrink when you gain and lose weight, but they don't change in number. Unlike some other cells, they do not regenerate. This means the results are relatively permanent in the suctioned area. If you do gain weight, then the liposuctioned area will never have the same bulk as it did before the surgery. Once the fat cells are gone from the area, they won't come back. However, if you gain weight, it will settle somewhere else.

### Who are the best candidates for liposuction?

The best candidates are people of normal weight who have excellent overlying skin tone, localized areas of fullness, and who realize liposuction is not a weight loss procedure. Age is less important, but older patients may not have the same skin elasticity as younger people.

### What happens in a liposuction procedure?

There are several different liposuction techniques, including tumescent, super-wet, power-assisted, vaser, and ultrasound-assisted lipoplasty. The procedure is generally done on a same-day basis, often in a surgical center specializing in cosmetic surgery, although high-volume procedures will need to be done in a hospital. Before surgery the areas to be suctioned will be marked with a marker-pen to ensure accuracy. In the surgery a narrow tube called a cannula is attached to a vacuum machine and is passed through small skin incisions, which are strategically placed in skin folds. A repetitive gliding and sucking motion removes tissue and sculpts the body into the desired contour.

**Is fat the only thing removed during liposuction?**

No. Fat isn't the only thing removed. Vital body fluids are removed as well, so it is important to replace these fluids to prevent shock.

**What happens after liposuction surgery?**

Most patients report pain is moderate to severe. Pain medication will be prescribed as will anti-nausea medication. Patients may experience burning, swelling, bleeding, and numbness. You can expect to feel stiff and sore for a few days. A snug elastic surgical garment is worn to control swelling for about six weeks following surgery. Swelling following the procedure may last up to six months, although many patients see a dramatic improvement within the first week. Bruising will improve within about three weeks and the areas of suction may feel numb and strange for a couple of months. Most people are able to return to work in about one week.

**What are the risks of liposuction?**

Although complications are rare, they do occur and include excessive fluid loss, friction burns, damage to the skin or nerves, and perforation injuries to vital organs. The most common problems are cosmetic and may cause irregular, asymmetric, or even baggy skin.

### Lower Body Lift

**What is a lower body lift?**

Patients who are not suited to liposuction alone may choose to have a lower body lift, which involves direct surgical excision of redundant skin and subcutaneous tissue. The procedure has many variations but generally involves a circumferential incision to remove excess abdominal, waist, buttock, and thigh tissue. A "total" body lift is an inpatient procedure and patients must be in excellent health to be suitable candidates. This procedure is becoming very common. Most of these patients have lost a large amount of weight due to stomach stapling procedures. Then the inelastic, over-stretched skin is left hanging after their massive weight loss.

### Thigh Lift

**What is a thigh lift?**

Thigh lifts were more frequent before liposuction techniques were introduced. The procedure is generally reserved for correcting skin laxity. The subcutaneous fat is suctioned and cut out from the inner and outer thighs. The procedure, risks, and complications are the same as those described for liposuction. The incisions are under tension, so there is more potential for wide scars.

### Upper Arm Lift

### What is an upper arm lift?

Upper arm lifts are not very common because liposuction can be used to treat the upper arm. Patients may be candidates for skin excision if they don't mind the scar and don't intend to expose their arms.

### New Treatments

### What are some new treatments?

Aging hands may develop dark brown or tan spots and the tissue over the back of the hand may thin. A new cream, Aldara, used in treating skin cancer has been found to rejuvenate sun-exposed skin and reduce the signs of age on the hands. Pulsed light treatment can be used to remove dark spots.

## PLASTIC SURGERY FOR MEN

### What percentage of men have plastic surgery?

Women have more plastic surgery than men do, although men receive 40 percent of all cosmetic ear surgery, 30 percent of rhinoplasty, and 90 percent of hair transplants. In addition, gynecomastia, or chest enlargement, deals exclusively with men.

### How can baldness be treated?

Incredible progress has been made in treating baldness. Re-establishing a hairline by rearranging the scalp hair pattern is now commonplace. Follicular unit transplantation involves using a dissecting stereomicroscope to divide naturally occurring follicular units from a donor strip of hair, giving natural-looking results.

### Can the eyes be treated?

The male upper eyelid is generally fuller than the female, and excess skin tends to appear more masculine. I'm always conservative in removing upper eyelid tissue in men as removing too much tissue will feminize the upper lid.

**What is gynecomastia?**

*Gynecomastia* is an enlargement of the breast in men. This condition is often hereditary and can cause great psychological discomfort. Overweight males tend to produce more estrogen, which also contributes to this problem. Most plastic surgeons use liposuction for this procedure as it achieves smooth outcomes.

**Is hair removal difficult?**

A current difficulty with hair removal is that multiple treatments are required for the average patient. Part of the problem is that hair growth involves three phases, so treatments are needed at various times to destroy the hair follicles in their different phases. There are many hair removal systems currently in use and most rely on damaging color cells in the hair bulb to destroy the hair.

**How do implants work in men?**

In men, facial implants are often placed to emphasize the jaw line, elevate cheekbones or lend prominence to a recessive chin. Other implants include pectoralis muscle implants, calf augmentation and buttock enhancement done with medical-grade elastomer prostheses.

**Can laser resurfacing be used on men?**

Because men don't use makeup, lasers are used rarely because of the risk of permanent skin color change. This is a serious concern when doing strong or deep laser treatments. Men's wrinkles tend to run deeper than women's because their skin is thicker, meaning stronger laser treatments are usually required.

**Is liposuction useful for men?**

For treatment of gynecomastia, ultrasound and power-assisted liposuction have been wonderful advances. Men also tend to see good results in reducing love handles around the waist and abdomen.

**Can men have browlifts?**

Brow placement is important in men because incorrect placement can feminize the face. I rarely perform forehead lifts on men and then only for extreme eyebrow droopiness, called ptosis, or when a patient has already undergone an upper eyelid tuck.

## What about facelifts?

Many surgeons modify the incisions when doing a male facelift and instruct their patients to let their hair grow out beforehand, so scars can be camouflaged by hair growth while they fade over the subsequent year. Male skin is thicker and doesn't lend itself to recontouring as easily as female skin, so a crisp neckline following a facelift can't always be achieved.

## How does a penile enlargement work?

Penile surgery can be done for either cosmetic or medical reasons. For cosmetic purposes, the ligaments that stabilize the base of the penis can be released with a surgical procedure, which lengthens the penis itself. Lipotransfer can also be used in the penile area to augment the size of the shaft. Removing an overhanging lower abdomen is another option, because although this will not make the penis longer it will certainly make it more visible.

A urologist can place penile implants for medical purposes. To form an erection, the man can inflate the implants from a pump located in the scrotum. Some men opt for surgical implantation of semi-rigid devices, although bendable silicone rods may be difficult to conceal because the penis remains permanently erect. Testicular implants made from pure silicone can also replace a testicle that has been lost.

## How does male rhinoplasty differ from female?

Most men come to my practice because of breathing problems due to previous nasal fractures. With male rhinoplasty patients, my goal is to balance the overall nose rather than reduce the underlying nasal structure too much.

## Can men have a tummy tuck?

Abdominoplasty for men emphasizes liposuction and, if necessary, skin excision rather than reinforcing the abdominal muscles. Men don't have their tummy muscles and skin stretched from pregnancy.


## REVISING PLASTIC SURGERY

### Why is revisional plastic surgery sometimes required?

I tell every patient who comes into my office that they may end up dissatisfied with their procedure and need revisional surgery. Every plastic surgeon occasionally has less than optimal results. Problems can occur for a number of reasons: Plastic surgery is an art and surgeons are working on the human body, which is a variable canvas; sometimes things just don't go as planned; and complications arise. Ideas of beauty are intangible, and a patient's concept of larger or smaller or prettier may not be the same as the surgeon's.

**What happens if I really dislike my surgery results?**

The best thing you can do is hang in there. Surgery can take a long time to heal – it might even take six months to a year before you can see the real results. Discuss your progress with your doctor at your follow-up visits and don't immediately start looking for a new surgeon. If you have done your homework and have chosen a qualified doctor to begin with, then trust that the doctor wants you to have the best possible result. Sticking with your original surgeon will also help you to keep your costs for revisional surgery down. If you have lost confidence in your original surgeon, then ask if he or she knows a colleague or trusted advisor available to give a second opinion. My advice is to keep your surgeon on your side, be willing to listen, and to remain calm if this happens.

## TAKING CARE OF YOUR SKIN

**What is the most important thing to consider when taking care of your skin?**

Avoiding the sun is the single most important action you can do to maintain a youthful appearance. UVA rays are the chief cause of wrinkling and cause the skin to take on a leathery appearance. UVA rays also cause sunspots, overall photo-aging changes, and the three types of skin cancers. UVB rays are most potent in causing sunburn and are considered to be the main cause of all three types of skin cancer.

**What is an SPF?**

Sun protection factor (SPF) measures the time a product protects against the skin reddening. If it takes 20 minutes for your skin to turn red in the sun, a sunscreen of SPF 15 allows 15 times the exposure. You should always wear a sunscreen of SPF 15 or higher and be sure whatever you use blocks both UVA and UVB rays. Sunblock is stronger than sunscreen. It physically deflects ultraviolet rays and is completely effective upon application.

**What ingredients should I look for in a sunblock?**

To block a substantial portion of UVA and UVB rays, look for a sunblock containing zinc oxide or titanium dioxide. If you sweat heavily look for a gel because they tend to stay on better than creams. Find a gel that contains Parsol or avobenzone.

**Is indoor tanning safe?**

No. Indoor tanning with or without burning causes photo-aging and an increased incidence of skin cancers.

**What does a good skin care program involve?**

Generally, a skin care program involves a cleanser followed by a conditioning solution that opens pores. If necessary, acne medication can be applied at this point. A vitamin C-based cell restorer can also be applied. Vitamin E also helps restore the skin, as well as directly protecting it from the harmful effects of solar radiation. Next, a rejuvenator such as Retin-A or copper peptides is applied, followed by sunscreen.

**What are some tips for maintaining youthful, healthy skin?**

To maintain youthful skin:
· Wear protective sunscreen or sunblock.
· Stay out of tanning booths.
· Do not smoke.
· Follow a regular skin care program.
· Maintain a healthy diet including whole grains, fruits, and vegetables.
· Exercise regularly.

**What treatments are available to enhance the skin?**

Although there are a multitude of skin treatments available, my favorites include Intense Pulsed Light (IPL) to blend sun-damaged color and citric acid or kojic acid peels for mild ongoing skin rejuvenation.

**How can I check for skin cancer?**

There are three general types of skin cancer:

*Basal cell carcinoma* usually has raised, pearly white edges and a depressed center. It may bleed and heal, bleed and re-heal.

*Squamous cell carcinoma*, which looks more like an ulcer or open sore, is more severe.

*Malignant melanoma* should be discovered early before it has time to spread around the body. Watch any skin lesions or growths for any type of change. Look for the three Bs—bigger, blacker, or bleeding—and if you notice any of them have a physician closely examine them. A suspicious attitude is a good thing when it comes to cancer.


## THE ZONE DIET

**What can I do if I'm worried about my weight?**

As a gift, I give my patients a book called *A Week in the Zone,* by Dr. Barry Sears. The book provides a simple method for choosing food and maintaining a healthy weight. You could also visit the website **www.drsears.com** for more information.

**What is *The Zone Diet?***

In *The Zone Diet* the quantity of food is less important than the quality. Carbohydrates are the culprits in driving insulin levels up and making the body an efficient fat-storing machine. *The Zone* is a balanced diet. It includes protein, carbohydrates, and fat, which are always eaten together.

*The Zone* includes consuming three meals and two snacks every day. In practical terms, you need to divide your meal plate into three equal sections and fill one section with a low-fat protein. You supplement this with vegetables and fruits and finally add a dash of healthy fat, such as olive oil, avocado, or slivered almonds. Consume few carbohydrates and eat regularly to maintain insulin levels.

*The Zone* diet purports to fight heart disease, diabetes, arthritis, fatigue, depression, cancer, hormone-related mood swings, multiple sclerosis, fibromyalgia, myriad disorders related to the inflammatory process. You don't need to be obsessive about it, just do the best you can. I believe you will soon feel healthier, have more energy, and be more alert.

## THE REST OF THE HEALTH AND BEAUTY PICTURE: DIET, EXERCISE, AND SKIN CARE

**What is the body mass index and why is it so important?**

Over the past ten years, the medical community has been replacing the old weight charts with a far more reliable tool: body mass index. The BMI measures the ratio of weight to size and takes into account those factors left out of the old charts. Your BMI is easy to calculate.

For the average adult a BMI under 18.5 is too thin. The normal range is 19–25. Overweight is 26–30, and anything over 30 is obese. You'll find BMI calculators on the Internet if you prefer not to do the math. The important thing is to monitor your BMI rather than your weight. Attention to BMI diverts your mind from the scale, which is psychologically healthy. Your BMI gives you a more accurate picture of your weight as an expression of fitness and self-care.

**What are antioxidants?**

In addition to a balanced intake of foods, we also need to be certain our diets provide a balance of vitamins and minerals. There is a special group of vitamins which are particularly important. These nutrients attach to non-nutritional elements in our bodies and prevent them from doing damage. These vitamins are called *antioxidants* since they attach to oxidized byproducts (free radicals) which can cause aging and disease in the body. Free radicals are also generated by sun exposure, smoking, and environmental pollutants. Some authorities believe food, rather than supplements, are a superior source of antioxidants. Make sure you eat plenty of fresh fruits and vegetables. The more colorful the pallette of fruits and vegetables, the more phytonutrients available.

**What are phytonutrients?**

*Phytonutrients* are a group of compounds that occur naturally in all the fruit and vegetables. They offer protection against cancer, heart disease, arthritis, hypertension, and other degenerative diseases. People who enjoy a diet rich in fruit and vegetables have a lower incidence of cancer, because these foods also protect against sun exposure, smoking, and environmental pollutants. Pumpkin is a perfect source for phytonutrients.

**Do people who exercise actually live longer?**

Yes. Compared to people who do not exercise, those who exercise regularly enjoy a longer lifespan and a better quality of life.

**Are anorexia and bulimia considered forms of dieting?**

No! Neither anorexia nor bulimia is a "diet." They are, instead, behavioral expressions of mental disorders and are best addressed by mental health practitioners and nutrition management. The people who deprive themselves of healthy nutrition in such extreme ways are engaged in a very deadly battle in which their lives are, quite literally, at stake. If you are attempting to starve your body to an unreasonable size and shape, I really encourage you to seek help and get yourself back in healthy control.

**What do you recommend for skin care?**

Personally I use a combination of vitamins A, C, and E, any available hydroxy acid gel, the moisturizing and nourishing natural plant-based Aveda skin care products (developed by Horst Rechelbacher), and a broad-spectrum sunscreen.

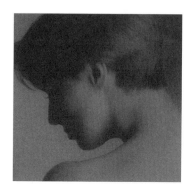

# GLOSSARY OF TERMS

# A

**Abdomen** – The part of the body cavity below the chest, separated by the diaphragm. The abdomen contains the organs of digestion and excretion. In women it also contains the uterus.

**Abdominoplasty** – Commonly known as a "tummy-tuck," this is a major procedure to remove excess skin and fat from the middle and lower abdomen and to tighten the muscles of the abdominal wall.

**Abscess** – A localized collection of pus that is usually infected and is caused by bacteria.

**Accutane** – Acne medication.

**Adipose tissue** – A complex layer of fat cells (adipocytes), connective tissue, and neurovasculature. This fibrous connective tissue occurs around the kidneys and in the buttocks. It serves both as an insulating layer and an energy store.

**Adrenaline** – A hormone secreted in the adrenal gland that raises blood pressure, produces a rapid heartbeat, and acts as a neurotransmitter when the body is subjected to stress or danger. The hormone epinephrine extracted from animals or prepared synthetically for medicinal purposes.

**Aesthetic surgery** – Surgery to alter or improve one's appearance.

**Aesthetic Surgery Journal** – Bi-monthly publication of the American Society for Aesthetic Plastic Surgery, providing articles on cosmetic procedures.

**Aesthetics** – The science that deduces the rules and principles of art. Concerned with beauty or the appreciation of beauty.

**Allergy** – A disorder in which the body becomes hypersensitive to particular antigens.

**Allograft** – Any human tissue that is transplanted from one body (usually a cadaver) to another. It is also called a homograft.

**Alphahydroxy acids (AHAs)** – Naturally occurring acids found in fruits and sugar cane.

**American Board of Medical Specialties (ABMS)** – This association approves medical training. The official surgery board for plastic surgeons is the American Board of Plastic Surgery.

**American Board of Plastic Surgery (ABPS)** – Certified plastic surgeons are members of this board. The ABPS is the only board approved by the American Board of Medical Specialties and the American Medical Association council for certifying physicians in plastic surgery.

**American Medical Association (AMA)** – This association is the largest association of medical doctors in the United States. Its purpose is to advance the interests of physicians, to promote public health, to lobby for medical legislation, and to raise money for medical education. The AMA also publishes the Journal of the American Medical Association (JAMA), runs the SAVE (Stop America's Violence Everywhere) program, and established the Council on Medical Education.

**American Society for Aesthetic Plastic Surgery (ASAPS)** – The leading professional society for plastic surgeons certified by the American Board of Plastic Surgery and seeking to further specialize in plastic surgery. The society's mission is to advance the science and art of cosmetic plastic surgery by supporting and directing education and research and by promoting the highest standards of ethical conduct and responsible patient care. It also provides information on plastic surgery to consumers.

**Analgesic** – A drug that relieves pain. Mild analgesics include aspirin and acetaminophen. More potent analgesics include hydrocodone and morphine.

**Anatomy** – The study of the structure and form of the various parts of the human body.

**Anchor incision** – An incision technique used in breast reduction and breast lift surgery. It forms a scar shaped like a boat anchor.

**Anesthesia** – A substance administered to a patient to cause a loss of sensation, especially pain, prior to a surgical procedure.

**Anesthesiologist** – A medically qualified physician who administers an anesthetic to induce unconsciousness in a patient prior to a surgical procedure.

**Angiogenesis** – The formation of new blood vessels as, for example, in an embryo or as a result of a tumor. It is promoted by growth factors.

**Antibiotic** – A substance, produced by or derived from a microorganism, that destroys or inhibits the growth of other microorganisms.

**Anti-inflammatory** – A substance known to counteract inflammation or swelling.

**Areola** – The naturally dark, round, pigmented area that surrounds the projecting nipple.

**Arm lift** – See *Brachioplasty*.

**Aspirin** – A drug widely used to relieve pain and to reduce inflammation and fever.

**Asymmetry** – Not symmetrical. When opposite parts of an organ or parts on opposite sides of the body do not correspond with each other in shape or size.

**Atherosclerosis** – Disease of the arteries in which fatty-tissue plaques develop on the inner surfaces of blood vessels. The plaques eventually obstruct blood flow.

**Autograft** – A tissue graft taken from the patient's own tissue. The graft is taken from one area of the body and is transferred to another part of the same individual.

**Avobenzone** – An ingredient found in sunscreen.

**Axilla** – The armpit or the cavity beneath the junction of the arm and shoulder.

# B

**Baldness** – Also called alopecia. The absence of hair, especially from the human head.

**Basal layer** – The bottom layer of skin.

**Beer belly** – A colloquial term commonly used to describe an extended stomach. Excessive beer drinking is not the only reason for the paunch, although this is a contributing factor.

**Belly button** – The umbilicus, commonly called a "navel" or "tummy button." It is essentially a scar caused by the removal of the umbilical cord.

**Bicep** – In general usage, bicep usually refers to biceps brachii, which is the prominent muscle on the upper arm.

**Blepharoplasty** – Cosmetic eyelid surgery.

**Board** – A medical specialty board certifies a particular branch of medicine. In regard to plastic surgery, the only official board that certifies a plastic surgeon is the American Board of Plastic Surgery.

**Body contouring** – In terms of cosmetic surgery, body contouring redefines the outline of the body. It is a term mainly used to describe liposuction.

**Botox injections** – Injections of Botulinum, a powerful nerve toxin produced by the bacterium Clostridium botulinum. Effective in minute doses for the treatment of muscle overreactions as it causes muscle paralysis.

**Bovine** – Of, or relating to, cattle. Some fillers are of bovine origin.

**Brachioplasty** – Also known as an arm lift, this operation reduces skin redundancy and fat volume, thereby improving the contour and shape of the upper arm. It invariably leaves a scar along the inner aspect of the arm.

**Breast augmentation** – A procedure to increase breast size. Implants are inserted subcutaneously to enlarge existing breast tissue.

**Breast crease** – The line or mark at the base of the breast, where the underwire of the bra would normally sit.

**Breast enlargement** – See *Breast augmentation.*

**Breast fold** – See *Breast crease.*

**Breast reconstruction** – The rebuilding of a breast or breasts that have been removed due to cancer or other disease.

**Breast reduction** – A procedure to decrease breast size.

**Breastbone** – Also called the *sternum.* A flat bone extending from the base of the neck to just below the diaphragm and forming the front part of the skeleton of the thorax. The breastbone articulates with the collarbones and the costal cartilages of the first seven pairs of ribs.

**Browlift** – A cosmetic procedure to elevate the area of the face in line with and above the eyes.

**Bruise** – An area of skin discoloration caused by the escape of blood from ruptured underlying vessels following injury.

**Burn** – An injury to the skin or tissue caused by heat, chemicals, radiation, or electricity. A first-degree burn affects the outer layer (epidermis) of skin, a second-degree burn affects both the epidermis and the underlying dermis, and a third-degree burn involves damage or destruction of the skin to its full depth and damage to the tissues underneath.

**Buttock crease** – Lower fold of the buttock.

**Buttock lift** – Surgery to remove excess fat from the buttocks.

# C

**Calcification** – Calcium deposits that form in the tissue around an implant, causing hardening and pain.

**Calf implants** – Implants used to enlarge the calf area.

**Cannula** – Long, thin, hollow, tubular instrument with side openings near one end and a connection to a high-pressure suction machine on the other, which is used to extract fat by vigorous back and forth motions during liposuction.

**Capsular contracture** – Scar tissue around a breast implant that causes pain, firmness, and sometimes a misshapen appearance.

**Carbohydrate** – Also called "carbs," this refers to a large group of organic compounds occurring in food and living tissues, including sugars, starch, and cellulose.

**Carcinoma** – A malignant growth; a cancer.

**Catheter** – A tube used for removing or injecting fluids into the body.

**Cartilage** – Cartilage is dense, connective tissue or gristle. It is a semi-opaque, grey or white in color, firm, flexible substance capable of withstanding considerable pressure.

**Cellulite** – A dimpled and irregular contour pattern of skin, thought to be due to the fatty deposits, toxins, and fluids trapped in pockets beneath the skin.

**Cheek implant** – A procedure in which a prosthesis is inserted into the lower region of the face in order to give the patient a higher cheekbone.

**Chemical peel** – Method of removing the superficial layer of skin by applying a caustic solution. This may also be called chemabrasion.

**Chin augmentation** – See *Genioplasty.*

**Chin implant** – The insertion of tissue or another object into the chin area of the face, so that the size of the chin is increased.

**Citric acid** – Soluble acid found in many fruits, particularly citrus fruits. Used in facial peels for ongoing skin rejuvenation.

**Cleft lip** – Also known as a hare lip, it is a congenital deformity of a cleft in the upper lip, on one or both sides of the midline. It occurs when three blocks of the embryonic tissue that form the upper lip fail to fuse and is often associated with a cleft palate. The medical name is cheiloschisis.

**Cleft palate** – An opening in the midline of the palate due to failure of the two sides to fuse in embryonic development. Only part of the palate may be affected, or the cleft may extend the full length with bilateral clefts at the front of the upper jaw bone. A cleft palate may be accompanied by a cleft lip and disturbance of tooth formation. The condition can be corrected with surgery.

**Collagen** – Fibrous insoluble protein found in connective tissue, extracted from cattle, from cadavers, or from the patient's own skin.

**Compression boots** – Used during some surgical procedures to prevent blood clots from forming.

**Congenital cup ear deformity** – An abnormality present at birth, in which the ears have not molded correctly. The condition can be fixed with otoplasty.

**Copper peptides** – A chain of amino acids used as an anti-aging formulation. It can also be used for healing wounds.

**Cortisone** – Originally a naturally occurring corticosteroid or hormone from the adrenal cortex, it is now prepared synthetically from Strophanthus or other plants, and is used in the treatment of arthritic ailments and many other diseases.

**Cosmetic surgeon** – A physician who has obtained a medical degree and specializes in cosmetic surgery.

**Cosmetic surgery** – Plastic surgery undertaken to improve the appearance.

**Cosmetic tattooing** – The act or practice of marking the skin with indelible ink to improve the appearance. The nipple can be tattooed onto the breast in a breast reconstruction.

**C-reactive protein (CRP)** – A nonspecific marker of inflammation. People with CRP in higher concentrations are more likely to have strokes, heart attacks, and vessel diseases.

**Crepey skin** – A wrinkled appearance, similar to crepe paper, in the skin.

# D

**Dead space** – The space created where an implant can be placed.

**Dehiscence** – The separation of the sutured edges of a surgical wound. It can be superficial (skin deep) or complete (down to the muscle fascia).

**Dermabrasion** – The removal or "sanding off" of the superficial layers of the skin with a rapidly revolving abrasive tool.

**Dermatologist** – A physician specializing in the skin, its structure, functions, and diseases, as well as its appendages such as the nails, hair, and sweat glands.

**Dermis** – The thicker layer of skin under the superficial epithelial cover called the epidermis. The hair follicles, sweat glands, blood vessels, and nerves reside in this deeper layer of skin.

**Diabetes** – An altered state of sugar metabolism due to insensitivity to insulin (type 2) or lack of insulin (type 1). Type 2 diabetes is common and leads to a variety of disorders of the cardiovascular system, nervous system, and skin. It is also called metabolic syndrome.

**Double bubble** – Occurs when there is a double fold at the bottom of the breast creating a "double bubble" appearance.

**Drain** – A plastic multiperforated tube, connected to a compressible vacuum bulb, which is placed under skin flaps to collect blood and serum.

# E

**Earlobe** – The lower, soft, fleshy part of the external ear.

**Echinacea** – A North American plant believed to stimulate the immune system and to ward off minor ailments such as cold and flu.

**Edema** – Swelling from an abnormal excess accumulation of watery fluid in connective tissue.

**Electrolyte** – A solution that produces ions. In medical terms it can also mean the ion itself. Concentrations of various electrolyte levels can be altered by many diseases, in which electrolytes are lost from the body (vomiting and diarrhea) or are not secreted (renal failure).

**Endoscope** – A small pencil-like camera that can be inserted through an incision to observe the inside of a hollow organ or body cavity.

**ENT** – See *Otolaryngology.*

**Enzyme** – A protein that acts as a catalyst (something that speeds up the rate of reaction without itself being used up in the reaction) of biological reactions.

**Enzyme system** – The body system responsible for transporting enzymes.

**Epidermis** – The superficial protective layer of skin overlying the dermis. The epidermis contains a maturing layer of epithelial cells including melanocytes, which impart color.

**Ethics** – Moral principles that govern people's behavior.

**Extrusion** – The erosion of skin that allows an implant to become exposed.

**Eyelid surgery** – See *Blepharoplasty.*

**Eyelid tuck** – See *Blepharoplasty.*

# F

**Facelift** – A cosmetic surgical procedure to lift and pull the face in an attempt to counteract the effects of aging and gravity.

**Facial plastic surgery** – Cosmetic surgery on areas of the face.

**Fascia** – The sheet of firm connective tissue that covers the muscles; sometimes used as graft material.

**Fascial system** – Supporting tissue layers on the body.

**Fat injection** – Taking fatty tissue from one area of the body and injecting it into another area.

**Fat suction** – Using pressure to remove or suck fat from areas of the body.

**Fat transfer** – Transferring fat from one region of the body to another.

**Fermentation** – The chemical breakdown of a substance by bacteria, yeast, and other microorganisms, typically involving release of heat.

**Fibromyalgia** – A disorder characterized by pain without inflammation in the fibrous tissue of the muscles. Widespread aching is usually accompanied by extreme fatigue and is often associated with headache, numbness, tingling, and other symptoms.

**Fillers** – Facial treatments injected into areas of the face in order to fill fine lines, wrinkles, and cheek folds. They can also be used for lip enhancement. Collagen and hyaluronic acid are common fillers.

**Forehead lift** – Surgery that tightens muscles and removes excess skin from the forehead.

# G

**Gallbladder** – A small pear-shaped organ lying underneath the right lobe of the liver. Bile is stored after secretion by the liver before release into the small intestine.

**General anesthesia** – A total loss of consciousness induced through inhalation of special gases or intravenous medication by an anesthetist or an anesthesiologist. Breathing is usually controlled through a tube placed in the airway. Supplemental intravenous narcotics and local anesthesia upon awakening reduce pain at the surgical site.

**General surgery** – Surgery of a non-specific nature.

**Genioplasty** – A cosmetic procedure to alter the size and shape of the chin by building it up with grafted bone, cartilage, or artificial material.

**Gingko** – An herbal product native to Asia believed to increase blood circulation and oxygen levels in the brain and in other critical organ tissues.

**Glaucoma** – A condition in which loss of vision occurs because of abnormally high pressure in the eye.

**Glycolic acid** – Fruit acid found in sugar cane.

**Graft** – Any organ, skin, or tissue used for transplantation to replace a faulty part of the body. In a skin graft, a healthy piece of skin is used to heal a damaged area of skin.

**Gynecomastia** – The development of female-like, enlarged breasts on a male. Its treatment is complicated by sagging, inelastic skin. Liposuction and chest wall skin excision are the common treatments.

# H

**Hematoma** – A collection of blood that forms in tissue, an organ, or body space as a result of persistent bleeding from injured blood vessels. An enlarging hematoma may be painful and must be evacuated by opening the nearby incision and removing the excess blood. Smaller hematomas are allowed to liquefy and sometimes are aspirated (suctioned with a needle placed through the skin) a week or so later.

**Hereditary** – Inherited characteristics. Traits passed on from one generation to another.

**Hibiclens** – (chlorhexidine) Antiseptic, antimicrobial skin cleanser.

**HMO manual** – A health-options manual for physicians.

**Hyaluronic acid** – Binding component of connective tissue.

**Hypertension** – Abnormally high arterial blood pressure, common in obesity. Leads to severe cardiovascular occlusive disease, kidney insufficiency, stroke, and premature death.

**Hypertrophic scar** – A thickened, elevated, red scar that fails to reduce in size over several months.

# I

**Immunology** – The study of immunity and all of the phenomena connected with the defense mechanisms of the body.

**Implant** – Tissue, or an artificial object, inserted into a person's body. Facial implants are often placed to emphasize the jaw line, elevate the cheekbones, and lend prominence to a recessive chin.

**Incision** – Cut made by a knife during surgery.

**Infection** – Invasion of the body by harmful organisms (pathogens).

**Intense Pulsed Light (IPL)** – A method of hair removal and skin rejuvenation by applying focused, broad-spectrum light to the surface of the skin by a hand-held wand or an articulated arm.

**Intravenous (IV)** – Within or into a vein.

**Involute** – Rolled inwards from the edge. Usually refers to the breast decreasing in size after child bearing.

# J

**Journal of Plastic and Reconstructive Surgery** – A monthly publication published by the American Society of Plastic Surgeons containing numerous articles on reconstructive and cosmetic procedures.

**Jowls** – Bulging laxity or fullness along the jaw lines lateral to the chin.

# L

**Laser** – An acronym for Light Amplification by Stimulated Emission of Radiation. An element usually made from carbon or erbium is used to emit radiation that is applied to the skin. Varied wavelengths are applied for a multitude of skin conditions.

**Laser resurfacing** – Involves applying a beam from a laser to the skin to alleviate wrinkles, acne, general scarring, age spots, brown spots, or sun-damaged skin.

**Laser safety officer (LSO)** – A person who inspects and approves the facility offering laser treatment.

**Lasik surgery** – A surgical procedure intended to reduce a person's dependency on glasses or contact lenses. It is used to correct both myopia (nearsightedness) and hyperopia (farsightedness).

**Laxity** – The quality or state of being loose.

**Lecithin** – One of a group of phospholipids that is an important constituent of cell membranes and is involved in the metabolism of fat by the liver.

**Lip augmentation** – Enlarging the size of the lips.

**Lipectomy** – Excision of fatty tissues.

**Lipoplasty** – See Liposuction.

**Lipostructure infiltration** – See *Fat injection*.

**Liposuction** – Technique for suctioning localized fat deposits from areas of the body such as the face, trunk, hips, and buttocks.

**Liposuction (high volume)** – Removing more than about five liters of subcutaneous tissue.

**Lipotransfer** – See *Fat injection*.

**Love handles** – Deposits of excess fat on the sides of a person's waistline.

**Lower body lift** – A procedure involving direct surgical excision of redundant skin and subcutaneous tissue of the waist, thighs, and buttocks.

# M

**MAC** – Stands for monitored anesthesia care.

**Malignancy** – The state or presence of cancer.

**Mammography** – An X-ray examination of the female breast. Fine details of breast tissue can be visualized, particularly the presence of calcification or soft tissue masses, enabling the early diagnosis of breast cancer.

**MAO inhibitor** – Monoamine oxidase (MAO) inhibitors are a class of drugs used for depression and Parkinson's disease. St. John's Wort is an MAO inhibitor that affects the enzyme system.

**Mastectomy** – Surgical removal of the breast.

**Mastopexy** – Breast lift procedure that improves the shape of the breast with nipple elevation.

**M.D.** – A doctor of medicine.

**Medical genetics** – The study of inheritance. It attempts to explain the inheritance of diseases throughout families.

**Melanoma** – A highly malignant form of skin cancer.

**Microfollicular grafts** – Hair follicle grafts used to treat baldness.

**Minimal incision facelift** – Also known as a short-scar facelift or a mini-lift, this procedure combines lipoplasty with less-invasive surgical procedures than those used in a traditional facelift.

**Minimally invasive surgery** – Operations performed through smaller incisions than in the past by the use of endoscopes, high-quality magnified video, and remote instrumentation.

**Mucosa** – Also called a mucous membrane, it is the membrane lining of many tubular structures and cavities, including the nasal sinuses, respiratory tract, gastrointestinal tract, and biliary and pancreatic systems.

# N

**Narcissist** – Someone who has an excessive or erotic interest in his or her self or his or her physical appearance.

**Nasal surgery** – See *Rhinoplasty*.

**Necrosis** – Tissue death usually due to inadequate blood supply.

**Neurotic** – Suffering from, or related to neurosis, which is a long-term mental or behavioral disorder in which contact with reality is abnormal. It features anxiety, phobias, and obsessions.

**Nicotine** – A poisonous alkaloid, nicotine is the active principle of tobacco and is the drug found in cigarettes.

**Nipple-areolar complex** – The nipple and the surrounding areola.

**Nonsurgical technique** – A cosmetic procedure that does not require surgery. Botox injections and laser resurfacing are examples of these techniques.

**Nose surgery** – See *Rhinoplasty*.

**No touch technique** – Also called *rapid-recovery breast augmentation*. This technique avoids touching the ribs during augmentation surgery.

**Nucleus** – The central or most important part of an object. In regard to cells, it is the part containing genetic material.

# O

**Orthopedic surgery** – Surgery for correcting deformities caused by disease of or damage to the bones and joints of the skeleton.

**Otolaryngology** – A branch of medicine concerned with the treatment and diagnosis of diseases of the ear, nose, and throat.

**Otoplasty** – Cosmetic ear surgery.

# P

**Pathology report** – A report based on microscopic evidence that describes cells and tissues. It is used to make a diagnosis of a disease.

**Pectoralis** – The large, flat muscle immediately under the breast that extends from the first seven ribs to the upper arm bone.

**Penile** – Relating to the penis.

**Perforation** – A hole made from piercing.

**Periareolar** – Around the areola. Refers to a concentric excision circle around the areola used in mastopexy.

**Periosteum** – A layer of dense connective tissue that surrounds all bones except those at the joints.

**Photo-aging** – Aging of the skin, mainly brought on by sun damage.

**Physical abnormality** – An irregularity in a person's appearance.

**Physician** – A registered medical practitioner or doctor who specializes in the diagnosis and treatment of disease.

**Physiology** – The branch of biology that deals with the normal functions of living organisms and their parts.

**Pixie ears** – Pointy, attached ears.

**Plastic surgeon** – A medical doctor who specializes in plastic surgery and who is certified by the American Board of Plastic Surgery.

**Plastic surgery** – Surgery that restores, repairs, or reconstructs body structure.

**Plasticos** – Greek word meaning *to shape, mold, or form.*

**Podiatrist** – A medical doctor specializing in treating the feet and associated ailments.

**Postoperative** – After the procedure or operation.

**Pressure bandage** – Material used to bind the wound and apply pressure, usually to stop a hemorrhage.

**Prophylactic** – An agent that prevents the development of a condition or disease.

**Prosthesis** – Artificial organ or part.

# R

**Radiology** – Branch of medicine involving the study of radiographs or other imaging technologies to diagnose or treat disease.

**Rapid-recovery breast augmentation** – See *No touch technique.*

**Reduction mammaplasty** – See *Breast reduction*.

**Reference** – A source of information used to ascertain something.

**Renova** – An anti-aging cream containing the active ingredient retinoic acid. It is said to lighten sunspots and reduce fine lines and wrinkles.

**Retin-A** – Trade name for *tretinoin*, a keratolytic agent used in the treatment of acne and sun-damaged skin.

**Revision** – Corrective or additional procedures on a previously operated-on site.

**Rhinoplasty** – *Rhino* means *nose*, and *plasty* means *to shape, mold, or form*. Plastic surgery of the nose.

# S

**Saddlebags** – The bulging and sagging skin along the upper, outer thighs in women.

**Salicylic acid** – A drug that causes the skin to peel and destroys bacteria and fungi.

**Saline** – Solution of salt and water.

**Scar** – A permanent mark left after a wound heals.

**Sclerotherapy** – Method of treating spider veins by injecting them with a corrosive solution.

**Sedative** – A drug that has a calming effect, relieving anxiety and tension.

**Shark cartilage supplement** – A supplement taken from a shark. Many people believe it can prevent or slow the formation of some cancers.

**Shock** – The condition associated with circulatory collapse, when the arterial blood pressure is too low to maintain an adequate supply of blood to the tissues.

**Silicone** – A chemical polymer of alternating silicone and oxygen atoms processed to a gel form to fill silicone elastomer breast implants.

**Skimmer** – A doctor who has not completed specialist training in plastic surgery yet performs cosmetic procedures.

**Sun protection factor (SPF)** – Measures the time a product protects your skin against sunburn. You should always use sunscreen with an SPF 15 or higher.

**State licensing** – A license that physicians must obtain from the state they wish to practice in.

**Subcutaneous** – Under the skin.

**Subcutaneous cells** – The cells found beneath the layer of skin.

**Subcutaneous fat** – The fat layer found under the skin. The layer cushions the dermis from underlying tissues such as muscle and bones.

**Subcutaneous tissue** – The variably thick composite connective and adipose tissue between the skin and the muscular fascia.

**Suction-assisted lipectomy** – Removal of fatty tissues via a suction machine.

**Surface work** – Other options available to people who want to enhance their appearance, without or in addition to surgery. Botox injections and chemical peels are examples of these options.

**Suture** – A strand or fiber used to sew together parts of the living body. Permanent sutures do not dissolve and absorbable sutures disappear in time. They are also known as stitches.

**Symptom** – A physical or mental feature that is regarded as indicating a disease.

# T

**Thigh lift** – Surgery to remove excess fat and skin from the thigh.

**Thoracic surgery** – Surgery to correct deformities or disease of the thorax or chest.

**Tissue-mimetic** – The imitation of tissue.

**Topical** – Applied to the skin.

**Torso** – The trunk of the human body, that is, the body excluding the head and limbs.

**Transconjunctival** – An internal incision of the lower eyelid to avoid an external scar.

**Trauma** – Physical injury or wound caused by external force or violence; an emotional or physical shock.

**Truncoplasty** – Molding or shaping the human torso. A body contouring technique, for example a buttock lift, can be combined with liposuction and a tummy tuck for a 360-degree truncoplasty.

**Tumescent technique** – Technique used in liposuction in which a solution of saline, a vasoconstrictor (vessel-constricting agent), and local anesthetic is injected into the tissues prior to suction.

**Tummy tuck** – See *Abdominoplasty*

# U

**Ultrasonic Assisted Lipoplasty** – The use of ultrasound technology to emulsify subcutaneous fat, sometimes followed by traditional liposuction.

**Upper arm lift** – Surgical procedure where skin is excised to improve an individual's cosmetic appearance.

**Urology** – Branch of medicine concerned with the functions and disorders of the urinary system.

# V

**Varicose veins** – Distended, swollen, knotted veins in the legs.

**Vascular structure** – Relating to or supplied with blood vessels.

**Vasodilator** – A drug that causes the widening of the blood vessels and therefore an increase in blood flow.

# W

**Wrinkling and folds** – Wrinkling or creasing of the breast implant surface that may result in visible irregularities.

# X

**Xenograft** – Treated animal tissue that can be used as a graft.

# Z

**Zinc oxide** – A skin protectant and wound healer. It is best to use a sunblock that contains this ingredient.

**Zone Diet** – A diet designed by Dr. Barry Sears, providing a simple method for choosing food and maintaining a healthy weight.

# References

Gryskiewicz, J.M. "Rhinoplasty: An Accurate Method to Trim the Lower Lateral Cartilages Through the Endonasal Approach." *Journal of Plastic and Reconstructive Surgery*, 92:344, 1993.

Rohrich, R.J. "Streamlining Cosmetic Surgery Patient Selection-Just Say No!" *Journal of Plastic and Reconstructive Surgery*, 104:220, 1999.

Gryskiewicz, J.M. "Recycling: Using the Distal Dorsum as a Sheen Graft." *Aesthetic Surgery Journal*, 20:457-464, 2000.

Gryskiewicz, J.M. "The 'Iatrogenic-Hanging Columella:' Preserving Columellar Contour After Tip Retroprojection." *Journal of Plastic and Reconstructive Surgery*, 110:272, 2002.

Gryskiewicz, J.M. Hatfield, A.S. "'Zigzag' Wavy-Line Periareolar Incision." *Journal of Plastic and Reconstructive Surgery*, 110:1778, 2002.

Gryskiewicz, J.M. "Submental Suction Assisted Lipectomy Without Platysmaplasty: Pushing the (Skin) Envelope to Avoid a Facelift in Unsuitable Candidates." *Journal of Plastic and Reconstructive Surgery*, 112:1393, 2003.

Gryskiewicz, J.M., Gryskiewicz, K.M. "Nasal Osteotomies: A Clinical Comparison of the Perforating Method Versus the Continuous Technique." *Journal of Plastic and Reconstructive Surgery*, 113(5):1445-1456, 2004.

# Index

Abdomen, described, 259
Abdominoplasty
    benefits of, 149, 154, 246–247
    candidates for, 149–150
    described, 259
    men and, 149, 177, 181, 252
    photographs of, 93, 153–160
    procedure, 150, 247
    recovery from, 152, 247
    revisional surgery for, 185–186
    risks associated with, 153, 247
    smoking and, 38
    types of, 150–152
Abscess, described, 259
Accutane, 145, 259
Acne scars, 190
Adipose tissue, described, 259
Adrenaline, described, 259
Advertising, false, 19–20
Aesthetic judgment
    body sculpting and, 148
    described, 13
    importance of, 5, 6
    liposuction and, 164
    photographs and, 52
    rhinoplasty and, 99, 238
Aesthetic surgery, described, 259
*Aesthetic Surgery Journal*, xii, 16, 259
Aging
    antioxidants and, 206, 209
    breasts and, 81
    browlift and, 127
    eyes and, 128, 134
    facelift and, 115, 124, 239–240
    facial changes from, 114
    fat loss and, 141
    gravity and, 5
    hand spots, 175, 250
    indoor tanning and, 198
    liposuction and, 164
    rapid phase of, 190
    skin tone and, 36
    sun and, 197
Alexis, Susan I., xii
Allergic reactions, 145
Allergy, described, 259
Allografts, 140, 269
Alphahydroxy acids (AHAs), 213–214, 260
American Board of Cosmetic Surgery, 14
American Board of Medical Specialties (ABMS)
    certification and, 12, 19, 225
    checking credentials with, 16
    overview of, 260
American Board of Plastic Surgery (ABPS)
    certification and, 19, 225
    checking credentials with, 16
    overview of, 13–14, 260

    physician referrals from, 22
American Medical Association (AMA)
    certification and, 19
    Council on Medical Education, 12, 225
    overview of, 260
American Society of Aesthetic Plastic Surgery (ASAPS)
    Gryskiewicz and, xi
    overview of, 15, 16–17, 260
    physician referrals from, 22
    requirements for election to, 227
    website of, 14, 20–21
American Society of Plastic Surgeons (ASPS)
    financing program of, 40, 41
    Gryskiewicz and, xi
    membership in, 226
    overview of, 15–16
    physician referrals from, 22
Analgesic, described, 260
Anatomy, defined, 260
Anchor incision, described, 261
Anesthesia
    for abdominoplasty, 150
    administrator of, 29, 229, 261
    for blepharoplasty, 135
    definition of, 261
    for facelift, 116
    for liposuction, 166–167
    types of, 232, 269
Anesthesiologist, described, 261
Angiogenesis, described, 261
Anorexia, 207, 257
Anti-inflammatory, described, 261
Antibiotic, described, 261
Antioxidant vitamins, 206, 209, 256
Areola, described, 261
Arm lift. See brachioplasty
Armpit breast augmentation photographs, 53, 68
Arthritis, 136
Aspirin, described, 261
Asymmetry, defined, 261
Atherosclerosis, described, 261
Atkins Diet, 217
Autografts, 140, 261
Avobenzone, 198, 262
Axilla, described, 262

Baldness
    described, 262
    treatments for, 177–178, 250
Basal cell carcinoma, 200, 254
Basal layer, described, 262
B.C. (Before Children) figure
    abdominoplasty for, 149, 246–247
    breast augmentation for, 51
    photographs of breasts, 55, 60, 62, 66
Beer belly, described, 262

Belly button, described, 262
Bicep, described, 262
Bilateral breast augmentation photographs, 57
Blepharoplasty
    associated procedures, 134
    benefits of, 128, 134, 138
    browlift instead of, 135
    men and, 177, 178, 250
    overview of, 243
    photographs of, 118–119, 121, 125, 130–133
    preparing for, 134–135
    procedure, 135–136
    recovery from, 136
    risks associated with, 136–137, 186–187
Blood pressure
    maintaining healthy, 211–212
    procedures and high, 124, 127, 136–137
Board certification
    checking, 16, 225–226, 227, 228
    confusion about, 14–15, 19
    importance of, 11–12, 183
    requirements, 12–14
Body contouring, described, 262
Body mass index (BMI), 203–204, 256
Body sculpting, 148
    See also specific procedures
Botox injections, 134, 143, 187, 246, 262
Bovine, described, 262
Brachioplasty, described, 262–263
Breast augmentation
    benefits of, 51, 232
    described, 263
    photographs of, 53, 55–70, 72–75, 77
    popularity of, 51
    procedure, 54–55, 71, 233
    recovery from, 56, 71, 75, 76, 78, 234
    revisional surgery rates for, 30
    risks associated with, 78–79, 187–188
    scars from, 20, 233, 234
    size of, 51–52, 54, 233
    See also implants, breast
Breast cancer
    breast reconstruction and, 87, 237
    implants and detection of, 54, 233, 234
Breast crease, described, 263
Breast enlargement. See breast augmentation
Breast enlargement in men, 178, 179, 191, 251,
    269
Breast-feeding, 51, 87, 90, 238
Breast lift. See mastopexy
Breast reconstruction
    benefits and timing of, 87
    breast cancer and, 237
    described, 263
Breast reduction
    benefits of, 237
    described, 263
    health insurance coverage for, 88–89
    photographs of, 91–92, 94–97
    procedure, 89–90, 237–238

    recovery from, 90, 238
    revisional surgery for, 188
    risks associated with, 90, 188, 238
    satisfaction with, 88, 89–90
Breastbone, described, 263
Brow-drop, 187
Browlift
    associated procedures, 134
    blepharoplasty instead of, 135
    described, 263
    men and, 177, 180, 251
    overview of, 124, 126
    photographs of, 118–119, 125, 132, 133
    procedure, 126, 241
    recovery from, 126, 241–242
    revisional surgery for, 188
    risks associated with, 188, 242
Bruise, described, 263
Bulimia, 207, 257
Burn, described, 263
Buttock crease, described, 263
Buttocks lift
    described, 247–248, 263
    with liposuction, 161
    photographs of, 174
    revisional surgery for, 189

C-reactive protein (CRP), described, 266
Calcification, described, 264
Calcification of breast implants, 79
Calf implants, described, 264
Cancers, 256
    See also breast cancer; skin cancers
Cannula, described, 264
Capsular contractures, 79, 264
Carbohydrates, 205–206, 217–218, 264
Carbon dioxide laser treatment, 146
Carcinoma, defined, 264
Cartilage, described, 264
Catheter, described, 264
Cellulite, described, 264
Cheek implants, 142, 189, 245–246, 264
Cheek lipotransfer, 118–119
Chemabrasion, 264
Chemical peels, 143–144, 177, 189, 246, 264
Chin augmentation, 138–139, 189, 244
Chin drop, 139
Chin implants
    described, 265
    for men, 179
    in modest chin augmentation, 244
    photographs of, 101, 104, 108, 125
    procedure, 138–139
    revisional surgery for, 189
Chin ptosis, 189
Citric acid, described, 265
Class reunion peel, 143–144
Classic abdominoplasty, 151–152
Classic mastopexy, 86
Cleft lip, described, 265

Cleft palate, described, 265
Closed rhinoplasty, 106
Cold sores, 145
Collagen, 198, 265
Collagen injections, 144, 145, 190, 246
Color step-off, 191
Communication with surgeon
    about expectations, 164, 165, 183, 185, 193
    dealing with complaints, 47
    dos and don'ts, 34–39, 229–230
    immediately prior to surgery, 55, 99
    instructions, 49
    *See also* consultations
Complaints, dealing with, 47
Complete abdominoplasty, 151–152
Compression boots, described, 265
Computer imaging, 33–34, 99, 229
Concentric mastopexy, 85–86
Congenital cup ear deformity, described, 265
Conrad, Joseph, 182
Consultations
    companion during, 35
    dos and don'ts, 34–39, 229–230
    fit with doctor, 25–27
    importance of, 183, 185
    initial, 228
    office staff and, 24–25
    overview of, 23–24, 37
    questions to ask during, 27–31
Contact lenses, 136
Copper peptides, described, 265
Cortisone, described, 265
Cosmetic ear surgery, 141–142
Cosmetic eyelid surgery. *See* blepharoplasty
Cosmetic surgeons
    described, 11–12, 226, 266
    meaningless certification, 14–15, 19
Cosmetic surgery, described, 266
Cosmetic tattooing, 140, 188, 266
Costs
    overview of, 40–42, 230–231
    reducing, 42
    for revisional surgery, 30, 184, 194
    *See also* health insurance coverage; payment
Credentials
    checking, 16, 225–226, 227, 228
    importance of, 11–12, 183
    meaningless, 14–15, 19
    specialty boards, 12–14
    training certificates, 29
Crepey skin, described, 266
Crescent mastopexy, 85

Dead space, described, 266
Dehiscence, described, 266
Dermabrasion
    associated procedures, 134
    described, 127–128, 242, 266
    photographs of, 118–119, 125
    repeat treatments, 190

Dermatologist, described, 266
Dermis, described, 266
Diabetes, described, 266
Diet
    cancer and, 256
    elements of good, 205–207
    food obsessions and needs, 204–205
    Gryskiewicz personal, 209–210, 211,
        212–213
    importance of, 203
    ORAC units, 209
    osteoporosis and, 207–208
    skin and, 200
    Zone Diet, 217–220, 255
Dog eared eyelids, 243
Dog ears, 137
Double bubble, described, 267
Doughnut mastopexy, 85–86
Drain, described, 267
Drooping eyebrows, 241, 243
Dry eye syndrome, 137, 186, 243
Dual-plane breast augmentation, 71, 72–75, 234
Ear surgery, cosmetic, 141–142, 245
Earlobe, described, 267
Eating disorders, 207, 257
Echinacea, described, 267
Edema, described, 267
Elastin, smoking damages, 198
Electrolyte, described, 267
Endoscope, described, 267
Endoscopic abdominoplasty, 149, 151
Endoscopic browlift, photographs of, 118–119,
    132
ENT. *See* otolaryngology
Enzyme, described, 267
Enzyme system, described, 267
Epidermis, described, 267
Epidural blocks, 167
Erbium laser treatment, 146
Ethics, described, 267
Exercise
    for abdominal area, 149
    after abdominoplasty, 152
    after breast augmentation, 75, 76
    after breast reduction, 90
    after browlift, 126
    after facelift, 123–124
    after liposuction, 167
    after mastopexy, 86, 87, 236
    elements of good program of, 208–209
    Gryskiewicz personal program of, 209–211
    importance of, 207–208, 257
    mental, 211
    skin and, 200
    types of, 207
Expectations
    from abdominoplasty, 150
    from cheek implants, 142
    communicating, 164, 165, 183, 185, 193

importance of realistic, 30, 35, 45–46, 186, 235

photographs and, 89–90, 128

when outcomes don't meet, 45–46

Extrusion, described, 267

Eyelid surgery. *See* blepharoplasty

Eyelid tuck. *See* blepharoplasty

Facelift

aging as reason for, 114–115

associated procedures, 134

avoiding tight look, 115–116

benefits of, 239

best candidates for, 115, 240

described, 268

men and, 177, 180, 252

minimal incision (mini-lift), 122, 123–124, 273

photographs of, 117–119, 122, 125

procedure, 116, 120, 240

recovery from, 124–125, 241

revisional surgery for, 190

risks associated with, 124, 241

signs of poor, 116, 240

smoking and, 38

Facial implants, 179

*See also* chin implants

Facial plastic surgery, described, 268

FACS, meaning of, 14

Family doctors, 22

Fascia, described, 268

Fascial system, described, 268

Fat, subcutaneous described, 277

Fat cells, 161, 164, 206, 217, 248

Fat injections

described, 268

for men, 180

overview of, 140–141, 245

photographs of, 125

revisional surgery for, 190

Fat suction, described, 268

Fat transfers. See fat injections

Fees. *See* costs

Fellow of the American College of Surgeons, 14

Fermentation, described, 268

Fibromyalgia, described, 268

Fillers, described, 268

Fish oils, 210, 211, 218–219

Food. *See* diet

Forehead lift, 268

*See also* browlift

Fredericks, Simon, xii

General anesthesia, described, 269

General surgery, described, 269

Genioplasty, 138, 244, 269

Gifts, 46

Gingko, described, 269

Glaucoma, described, 269

Glycolic acid, described, 269

Grafts, 139–140, 269

Gravity, 5, 81, 87, 114

Gryskiewicz, Joe

background of, xi–xii, 13

honors and awards received by, xii

personal health program of, 209–213

personal skin care program of, 214

photographs of, xiii

volunteer work by, xii

website of, 8, 21, 54, 224

Gynecomastia, 178, 179, 191, 251, 269

Hair removal, 178–179, 251

Hair transplantation, 177, 188, 190, 191

Hand rejuvenation, 175

Happy Patient Lists, 21

Hare lip, described, 265

Health insurance coverage

for blepharoplasty, 128

for breast reconstruction, 87

for breast reduction, 88–89, 237

for otoplasty, 142

restrictions on, 11, 42–43, 231, 270

for rhinoplasty, 181

Hematoma, described, 269

Herbals, 37, 124

Hereditary, described, 270

Herpes, 145

Hesperidin, 210

Hibiclens, described, 270

High blood pressure, 124, 127, 136–137, 270

Hips, 162

HMO manual, described, 270

Homografts. *See* allografts

Hospital privileges, 11, 28–29, 226

Hyaluronic acid fillers, 144, 145, 246, 270

Hypertension, described, 270

Hypertrophic scars, 195, 270

Immunology, described, 270

Implants, breast

complications with, 30, 70, 78–79, 187, 235

mammography and, 54, 233, 234

mastopexy and, 80

photographs of, 77

size of, 51–52, 54, 233

types of, 54, 233

Implants, cheek, 142, 189, 245–246

Implants, chin

for men, 179

photographs of, 101, 104, 125

procedure, 138–139, 244

revisional surgery for, 189

Implants, described, 270

Implants for men, 179, 181, 251, 252

Incisions

in abdominoplasty, 149, 151, 152, 153, 159

in blepharoplasty, 135, 136, 137

in breast augmentation, 54–55

in browlift, 126

in chin augmentation, 138
described, 270
in facelift, 116, 120, 123, 180
in mastopexy, 85, 86, 87, 236
in mid-face lift, 127
in thigh lift, 170
types of, 261
Indoor tanning, 198, 254
Infection, described, 270
Information sources
about area plastic surgeons, 16, 22, 227
about breast augmentation, 54
about plastic surgery, 7, 8, 14, 20–21, 224
about Zone Diet, 217, 255
Insurance coverage. *See* health insurance coverage
Intense Pulsed Light (IPL) treatments, 200, 254, 270
Internal (breast) lift, 234
*See also* dual-plane breast augmentation
International Society of Clinical Plastic Surgeons, xi
Intravenous (IV), described, 270
Intravenous (IV) sedation, 166
Involute, defined, 271

*Journal of Plastic and Reconstructive Surgery*, xii, 16, 271
Jowls, 114, 271

Laser, defined, 271
Laser safety officer (LSO), described, 271
Laser skin resurfacing
described, 271
for hand rejuvenation, 175
for men, 179, 251
overview of, 145–147, 246
revisional surgery for, 191
Laser surgery, 134
Lasik surgery, described, 271
Laxity, defined, 271
Lecithin, 37, 271
Leg vein treatments, 175, 191
LeGuin, Ursula K., 4
Limited abdominoplasty, 151
Lip augmentation, surgical, 139–140, 191–192, 244–245, 271
Lipectomy, described, 271
Lipoplasty. *See* liposuction
Lipostructure infiltration. *See* fat injections
Liposuction
abdominoplasty and, 150, 151
associated procedures, 161, 165, 169–170, 238, 247
benefits of, 164–165, 169, 248
best candidates for, 164, 248
communicating expectations about, 164, 165
described, 272, 278
high volume of, 272
limitations of, 36
for men, 177, 178, 179, 181, 251
on neck, 120, 121, 192, 240

overview of, 161
photographs of, 93, 121, 160, 162–163, 171
procedure, 165–167, 248
recovery from, 167–168, 249
revisional surgery for, 192
risks associated with, 39–40, 166, 168–169, 192, 249
on thighs, 93, 160, 162–163, 169–170, 192
on upper arms, 170, 171, 195
Lipotransfer. *See* fat injections
Love handles, described, 272
Lower body lift, 169, 249
Lunch-hour peel, 143

MAC, 166, 272
Malignancy, described, 272
Mammography, 54, 78, 233, 234, 272
MAO inhibitor, described, 272
Mastectomy
breast reconstruction after, 87, 237
described, 272
Mastopexy
benefits of, 235
described, 272
overview of, 80–81, 235
photographs of, 81–84, 85, 172
procedure, 85–86, 236
recovery from, 85, 86–87, 236
revisional surgery for, 188
risks associated with, 87, 236
Medical genetics, described, 273
Medical history
importance of being honest about, 30, 36–37, 230
relation of risks to your, 28, 30
Medical specialty board, described, 262
Melanomas, 200–201, 255, 273
Men, plastic surgery and, 149, 177–181, 191, 250–252
Microfollicular grafts, described, 273
Mid-face lift, 127, 129, 190, 242
Mini-lift (minimal incision facelift), 122, 123–124, 240, 273
Minimally invasive surgery, described, 273
Modified abdominoplasty, 151
Moles, 201
Monitored anesthesia care (MAC), 166, 272
Monkey lip profile, 140
Mucosa, 273

Narcissists, 46, 273
Nasal surgery. *See* rhinoplasty
Neck liposuction (without facelift), 120, 121, 192, 240
Necrosis, described, 273
Neurotic, described, 273
Nicotine use
being honest about, 38
effect on procedures of, 90, 124, 230
nicotine defined, 273

skin and, 198–199

Nipples
    breast reduction and, 88, 89, 90
    correcting inverted, 65
    mastopexy and, 80, 81, 85–86, 235
    postoperative numbness, 78, 188, 235, 238
No-touch technique, 71, 234, 275
Nonsurgical technique, described, 274
Nose reshaping. *See* rhinoplasty
Nucleus, described, 274

On-line information
    about area plastic surgeons, 16, 22, 227
    about breast augmentation, 54
    about plastic surgery, 7, 8, 14, 20–21, 224
    about Zone Diet, 217, 255
Open rhinoplasty, 104–106
Orthopedic surgery, described, 274
Osteoporosis, 207–208
Otolaryngology, described, 274
Otoplasty
    described, 274
    men and, 177
    overview of, 141–142, 245
    revisional surgery for, 193
Oxygen Radical Absorbance Capacity (ORAC)
    values, 209

Parsol, 198
Pasta diet, 204
Pathology report, described, 274
Patient coordinators, 25
Payment
    for breast reduction, 88–89, 237
    common practices, 40–41, 231
    financing from ASPS, 40, 41
    for otoplasty, 142
    *See also* health insurance coverage
Pectoralis, described, 274
Penile, defined, 274
Penile enlargement, 180–181, 252
Penile implants, 181, 252
Perforation, defined, 274
Periareolar, described, 274
Periosteum, described, 274
Photo-aging, described, 275
Photographs
    from computer imaging, 33–34
    of desired results, 34–35, 80, 99
    expectations and, 89–90, 128
    of prior patients, 29, 237
    using in breast augmentation, 52
    using in breast reduction, 89–90
    *See also under specific procedures*
Physical abnormalities, correcting, 6
Physical abnormalities, described, 275
Physical activity. See exercise
Physician, defined, 275
Physiology, defined, 275
Phytonutrients, 256

Pixie ears, 275
Plastic surgeons
    choosing, 184, 226, 227–228
    described, 275
    finding, 21–24, 227–228
    information about, 22–23
    instructions from, 49
    professional organizations for, 15–17
    qualities of good, 8–9
    relationship with, 45–47, 231
    specialty training of, 12–14
    trust in, 33
    *See also* credentials
Plastic surgery
    described, 275
    goals of, 5–7, 223
    public opinion about, 5
    reasons not to have, 8–9, 35, 225
Plastic surgery junkies, 46
Podiatrist, described, 275
Postoperative, defined, 275
Power-assisted liposuction, 179
Pre-pregnancy figure.
    *See* B.C. (Before Children) figure
Pregnancy
    abdominoplasty and, 149–150
    mastopexy and, 80, 236
Prescription medicines. See medical history
Pressure bandage, described, 275
Privacy, 28
Private office surgeries, 11
Procedures
    combining, 134, 141, 161, 165, 169–170,
        238, 247
    demographics of, 5, 223
    length and risks involved, 39
    locations of, 11, 28–29, 228–229
    number annually, 39, 223
    *See also specific procedures*
Professional organizations, 15–17, 22–23
Prophylactic, described, 275
Prosthesis, described, 275
Protein, 210, 218–219
Pseudobursa, 185
Ptosis, 180, 189, 251
Pulsed light treatment, 250

Qualifications. *See* credentials

Radiology, defined, 275
Rapid-recovery breast augmentation, 71, 234, 275
Recommendations, 21–24, 227–228
Reconstructive surgery, 12–13, 42
Recovery
    from abdominoplasty, 152, 247
    activity restrictions during, 31
    from blepharoplasty, 136
    from breast augmentation, 56, 71, 75, 76, 78,
        234
    from breast reduction, 90, 238

from browlift, 126, 241–242
from chin augmentation, 139
depression during, 232
from facelift, 123–124, 241
from laser skin resurfacing, 146
from liposuction, 167–168, 249
from mastopexy, 85, 86–87, 236
from mid-face lift, 127
revisional surgery and, 183, 253
from rhinoplasty, 100, 239
Reduction mammoplasty. *See* breast reduction
Reference, defined, 276
Renova, described, 276
Retin-A, described, 276
Revisional surgery
for abdominoplasty, 185–186
after liposuction, 169
for blepharoplasty, 186–187
for breast augmentation, 187–188
for breast reduction, 188, 191
for browlift, 188
for buttocks lift, 189
for cheek implants, 189
for chin augmentation, 189
costs of, 184
for facelift, 190
for leg vein treatments, 191
for lip augmentation, 191–192
for liposuction, 192
for mastopexy, 188
for otoplasty, 193
policy on, 28, 30, 229
reasons for, 183, 186, 252–253
for rhinoplasty, 30, 99, 194–195, 239
for scars, 195
for thigh lift, 195
timing of, 183
for upper arm lift, 195
Rhinoplasty
closed, 106
cost of, 194
described, 276
frequency of, 238
men and, 177, 181, 252
open, 104–106
overview of, 99–100
photographs of, 101–104, 106–112
procedure, 100, 239
recovery from, 100, 239
revisional surgery for, 30, 99, 194–195, 239
risks associated with, 113, 239
success of, 238–239
Rhinoplasty Society, xi
Rohrich, Rod J., 44

Saddlebags, described, 276
Salicylic acid, described, 276
Saline, described, 276
Saline implants, 54, 77, 78, 233
Scars

from abdominoplasty, 149, 152, 153, 246
from acne, 190
from blepharoplasty, 135, 136, 243
from breast augmentation, 71, 76, 233, 234
from breast procedures, 188
from breast reduction, 89, 90, 95, 97,
237–238
from browlift, 126, 188
from buttocks lift, 161, 189
from chin augmentation, 138
defined, 276
from facelift, 123, 180, 190, 240
hypertrophic, described, 270
from liposuction, 168, 169
from mastopexy, 81, 85, 86, 87
necessity of, 20
from otoplasty, 193
permanency of, 19
from revisional abdominoplasty, 185
revisional surgery for, 195
from thigh lift, 250
from upper arm lift, 170, 195
Sclerotherapy, 175
Sears, Barry, 205, 210, 216–220, 255
Second-hand smoke, 38, 90, 124
Sedative, described, 276
Self-esteem, 5, 6, 141–142, 223
Septal perforations, 194
Shark cartilage supplement, described, 276
Shock, described, 276
Short scar facelift, 122, 123–124
Silicone, described, 277
Silicone implants, 54, 233
Skimmers, 12, 226, 277
Skin
crepey, 266
maintaining youthful, healthy, 197–200,
213–214, 253–254, 257
*See also* wrinkles
Skin cancers
indoor tanning and, 198
sun and, 197, 253
types of, 200–201, 254–255
Skin care, 253–255
Smoking
abdominoplasty and, 153, 185
being honest about, 38, 230
breast reduction and, 90
effects on procedure outcomes and, 230
facelift and, 124
leg vein treatments and, 191
skin and, 198–199
Specialty boards. *See* board certification
SPF (sun protection factor), 197, 253, 277
Sports drinks, 212
Squamous cell cancer, 200, 255
Stallone, Sylvester, 176
State licensing, described, 277
State medical boards, 23, 225
Stomach surgery. See abdominoplasty

Subcutaneous, described, 277
Subcuticular sutures, 136
Suction-assisted lipectomy, described, 277
Sun
    after browlift, 126
    after facelift, 123
    after liposuction, 168
    skin and, 197–198, 199, 253
    spots from, 250
    treatment for skin damaged by, 254
Sunscreens and sunblocks, 197–198, 199,
    253–254
    Supplements
    benefits from, 206
    potential problems from, 37
    for skin care, 257
    taken by Gryskiewicz, 210
Surface work
    Botox injections, 134, 143, 187
    chemical peels, 143–144, 177, 189
    collagen injections, 144–145, 190
    described, 246, 277
    laser skin resurfacing, 145–147, 246
    tissue fillers, 144–145
Surgery centers, 11, 165
Surgical lip augmentation, 139–140
Surgical revisions. See revisional surgery
Sutures, described, 277
Symptoms, described, 277

Tanning, 197–198, 253–254
Tear production, 134, 186
Tebbetts, John, 32
Testicular implants, 181, 252
Thigh lift
    described, 278
    overview of, 169–170, 249–250
    photographs of, 173–174
    revisional surgery for, 195
Thigh liposuction photographs, 93, 160, 162–163
Thoracic surgery, described, 278
Thyroid disease, 136
Tissue, subcutaneous, described, 277
Tissue fillers, 144–145, 246
Tissue-mimetic, described, 278
Titanium dioxide, 197, 254
Topical, described, 278
Torso, defined, 278
Total body lift, 249
Training certificates, 29
Trans-fatty acids, 210
Transconjunctival incisions, 135, 278
Trauma, described, 278
Truncoplasty, 248, 278
Tumescent technique, described, 278
Tummy tuck. See abdominoplasty

Ultrasonic assisted lipoplasty, 278
Ultrasound-assisted liposuction (UAL), 166, 179
Ultraviolet-A (UVA) rays, 197, 198, 253

Ultraviolet-B (UVB) rays, 197, 198, 253
Upper arm lift
    described, 250, 278
    overview of, 170
    photographs of, 172, 174
    revisional surgery for, 195
Urology, defined, 279

Varicose veins, described, 279
Vascular structure, defined, 279
Vasodilator, described, 279
Vein treatments, 175
Vitamins
    antioxidants, 206, 209, 256
    for skin care, 199, 200

Walking, 167
Water, drinking, 211, 212–213
Websites. See on-line information
Week in the Zone, A (Sears), 217, 255
Weight
    abdominoplasty and, 149, 246–247
    BMI and, 203–204, 256
    body lift and, 249
    breasts and, 81, 188
    gynecomastia and, 178
    ideal, 203–204
    liposuction and, 164
    lower body lift and, 169
    total body lift and, 172–174
Witch's chin, 139, 244
Wrinkles
    Botox injections and, 134, 143, 246
    breast implants and, 79, 279
    chemical peels and, 143–144, 246
    collagen injections and, 144–145, 246
    fat injections and, 245
    laser skin resurfacing for, 145–147
    men and, 179, 251
    preventing, 213–214
    from sun, 253

Xenografts, 140, 279

Yellow Pages, 19
Yo-yo diet syndrome, 217

Zinc oxide, 197, 254, 279
Zone Diet, The (Sears), 205, 216–220, 255, 279